LEGAL ISSUES IN HUMAN REPRODUCTION

Forthcoming titles in the series:

New Reproductive Techniques: A Legal Perspective
Douglas J. Cusine, University of Aberdeen

A Patient's Right to Know: Information, Disclosure, the Doctor and the Law
Sheila A. M. McLean, University of Glasgow

Medico-Legal Aspects of Reproduction and Parenthood
J. K. Mason, University of Edinburgh

Law Reform and Human Reproduction
Edited by *Sheila A. M. McLean*, University of Glasgow

Legal and Ethical Issues in the Management of the Dementing Elderly
Mary Gilhooly, University of Glasgow

Discrimination and Mental Illness
Tom Campbell, University of Glasgow and *Chris Heginbotham*, King's Fund College

Pharmaceuticals in the European Community
Ken Collins, Member of the European Parliament and *Sheila A. M. McLean*, University of Glasgow

Pregnancy at Work
Noreen Burrows, University of Glasgow

Changing People: The Law and Ethics of Behaviour Modification
Alexander McCall Smith, University of Edinburgh

The Law and Economics of Health Care Allocation
R. Lee, University of Lancaster

Surrogacy and the Moral Economy
Derek Morgan, University College, Swansea

The Right to Reproduce and the Right to Found a Family
Athena Liu, University of Hong Kong

Family Planning and the Law
Kenneth Norrie, University of Aberdeen

Mental Health Law in Context: Doctors' Orders?
Michael Cavadino, University of Sheffield

The Changing Nature of Medical Autonomy
Leanna Darvall, La Trobe University

All titles are provisional

LEGAL ISSUES IN HUMAN REPRODUCTION

Edited by
SHEILA McLEAN

Dartmouth

Aldershot · Brookfield USA · Hong Kong · Singapore · Sydney

Published by
Dartmouth Publishing Company Limited
Gower House
Croft Road
Aldershot
Hants GU11 3HR
England

Gower Publishing Company
Old Post Road
Brookfield
Vermont 05036
USA

Library of Congress Cataloging-in-Publication Data
Legal issues in human reproduction/edited by Sheila McLean.
     p. cm.—(Medico–legal issues; v.)
  Bibliography: p.
  Includes index.
  1. Human reproduction—Law and legislation. I. McLean,
Sheila. II. Series.
  K2000.L44 1989
  344'.0419—dc19
  [342.4419]   88–25199
                                              CIP

British Library Cataloguing in Publication Data

Legal issues in human reproduction.—
  (Medico–Legal issues).
  1. Man. Reproduction. Legal aspects
  I. McLean, Sheila A.M. II. Series
  342.4'419

ISBN 1 85521 008 8

Printed and bound in Great Britain by
Courier International Ltd, Tiptree, Essex

Contents

Acknowledgements

Firstly, I am of course extremely indebted to the distinguished contributors to this volume for the time, thought and energy which they have put into their chapters. I hope that the readers learn as much from their contributions as I did!

Inevitably, the collection and preparation of a manuscript such as this is time-consuming, and I am deeply indebted to my Head of Department, Professor Alan Watson, for his patience and understanding in the face of the inroads made into my departmental time, and for his constant interest and support. Liz Doherty was, as ever, an invaluable colleague and without her excellent typing and willing assistance, life would have been much harder. John Irwin and the staff at Gower have been their usual constructive and considerate selves, for which I thank them. And finally, but importantly, I must record a great and continuing debt to my family and friends for their encouragement and support.

Sheila McLean

Contributors

Rebecca Cook is Professor of Law at the University of Toronto.

Douglas Cusine is Senior Lecturer in Law at the University of Aberdeen.

Bernard Dickens is Professor of Law at the University of Toronto.

Michael Freeman is Professor of English Law at the University College, London.

Christopher Heginbotham is National Director of the National Association for Mental Health [MIND].

Michael Kirby is President of the Supreme Court, New South Wales.

Ken Mason is Emeritus Professor of Forensic Medicine at the University of Edinburgh.

Sheila McLean is Director of the Institute of Law and Ethics in Medicine, University of Glasgow.

David Meyers is an attorney in California.

Introduction

Human reproduction is a matter of perennial public interest and debate. Modern reproductive methods and techniques have added increased complexity to this debate, whilst removing none of the original issues of concern.

Inevitably, given the complexity of the subject, it is not possible to be completely comprehensive of all the issues and, as the title of this book suggests, a number of them – some new and some less so – have been selected for consideration here. Although some contentious issues, such as embryo experimentation, are not therefore directly tackled, it is hoped that the topics chosen represent a reasonable sampling of the various relevant interests, and that they can provide some insights which reach beyond the actual title of the chapters themselves. Rather than being simply a statement of the nature of certain problems, this book is designed to tease out and analyse some of the fundamental issues raised by traditional and innovative reproductive practices, and to consider the implications of technological advance for the fertile and the infertile, embryos and foetuses, children and women. Given the seemingly inexhaustible supply of potential topics, the inevitable diversity of views and the differences in the types of problems posed, no attempt has been made to impose a general theme or approach on contributors. Thus, the book contains – as it was designed to do – a variety of viewpoints. This is seen as a benefit in a book of this nature, since our aim is not to impose by academic argument a seemingly incontrovertible logic on these highly sensitive matters, nor to discredit genuinely held views. Rather, the book is designed to give an international and interdisciplinary insight into some of the possible mechanisms for resolution of disputes and debates, and it is hoped, therefore, that whether or not the reader finds his or her particular approach represented here, each contribution will stimulate constructive comment and consideration of these important and controversial matters, and will whet the reader's appetite for the books to follow in this series.

The law as stated is, as far as possible, accurate to January 1988.

Sheila A. M. McLean,
The University of Glasgow,
March 1988.

1 Medical technology and new frontiers of family law*

MICHAEL KIRBY

In the rear and limping

In *Mount. Isa Mines Limited* v. *Pusey*[1] Windeyer, Justice of the High Court of Australia wrote of 'law, marching with medicine but in the rear and limping a little . . .'.[2] This remark, addressed to the stumbling approach of the law to the provision of damages for nervous shock occasioned by negligence, may be too kind when applied to the response of family law to the remarkable advances of knowledge and technology affecting human sexuality and conception.

Nowadays there is a growing sense of urgency and impatience about the response of the law to medical developments. One writer trained both in law and medicine observed from an informed standpoint:

> Those doctors who have studied law have always been uneasy at the extent to which Anglo-Saxon law departs from reality in dealing with biological issues. The nervous shock cases which continue to be based on medical principles discarded during the 19th century provide a notorious example. The irreconcileable differences between the legal concept of criminal responsibility and the actual behaviour of offenders who suffer from mental disorder, the bizarre principles by which conviction and punishment are meted out to those accused of what is considered to be irregular sexual behaviour, are fully appreciated only by those doctors who choose to appear as expert witnesses, or who come into contact with the accused persons.[3]

To these cases for anxiety and impatience must now be added the impact of the developments concerning human procreation and conception as affecting family law. Numerous international human rights statements declare the family to be the natural unit for the organization of human society.[4] Although, in many countries, changes have occurred in conceptions of marriage and the family – many of them consequent upon advances in the status of women, the sexual revolution, developments in contraception and other economic and social changes – the forces which promote the cohabitation of men and women remain basically the same. They include the achievement of sexual satisfaction, the procreation of children and congenial companionship. The law has changed in many jurisdictions to reflect changes which have occurred in attitudes to marriage, the family and the children of such relationships. For example, there have been important changes in the family law of many Commonwealth countries, responding originally to a report of the (English) Law Commission[5] which proposed the replacement of matrimonial fault as a ground for dissolution of marriage by the consensual principle addressed to the irreconcilable breakdown of the relationship.[6] In some countries, however, and in many US states it is still necessary to prove a matrimonial offence. Under that regime, adultery remains one of the principal grounds of divorce. Other typical changes in family law have been the adoption of new laws on illegitimate or ex-nuptial children[7] and, more recently, new laws on *de facto* relationships.[8]

Abnormal conception

For millennia, the normal method of securing human conception has been by sexual intercourse between man and woman, who might or might not be married. It was to the consequences of the conception, rather than the mode of its attainment, that that area of law now called family law was typically addressed. It is only in recent years that medical technology has refined conception by artificial insemination. Still more recent are the developments of *in vitro* fertilization and surrogate births. Most recent of all is the procedure called 'gamete intra-fallopian transfer'.[9]

It may be useful to describe briefly each of these new techniques. It is important to recognize that, in each of them, the overwhelming problem being addressed is infertility – that is, the inability of the couple to secure conception by sexual intercourse. Despite occasional reports of homosexual partners who resort to the procedures to avoid heterosexual intercourse, the significant problem is overwhelmingly one of persons in a heterosexual relationship (most of them married) who discover that the relationship is involuntarily infertile. Although there are no accurate figures on the extent of infertility, it is widely stated that some 10 – 15 per cent of marriages fall into this class.[10]

The oldest techniques to overcome infertility, in use for several decades, are artificial insemination by husband (AIH) and artificial insemination by donor (AID). There is relatively little opposition to AIH, although some religions cannot countenance it because of the separation of the 'unitive' and procreative aspects of sexual intercourse.[11] Much more controversial is AID, which is said to produce some 2,000 to 4,000 births per year in the United Kingdom alone.[12] AID is typically adopted where the husband's semen is inadequate in quantity or quality. The couple are counselled. The anonymous donor then becomes the genetic father of the child even though the partner (husband) will become its social father, in the sense of providing security and affection to the child so produced. The identity of the genetic father is typically withheld. In the United Kingdom and Australia it seems that medical students are often used as volunteers. Other fertile men may also be used as donors, raising the question of whether they should have the informed consent of their wives.[13] To avoid the risk of incestuous union between AID children, it has been suggested that administrative controls should limit the number of inseminations from the same donor. Figures ranging from 5 to 20 are mentioned.[14]

In 1984 the *Report of the Committee of Inquiry into Human Fertilisation and Embryology* (the Warnock Report)[15] recommended legislative changes in the United Kingdom designed to incorporate the child born by AID procedures into the family and to equate such a child to a child of the marriage. The Committee unanimously recommended that the AID child should be treated in law as the legitimate child of its mother and her husband in cases where they have both consented to the treatment.[16] It recommended a change in the law to clarify the fact that the semen donor would have no parental rights or duties in relation to the child. But it also recommended that, on reaching the age of 18, the child should have access to the basic information about the donor's ethnic origin and genetic health and that legislation should be enacted to provide the right of access to this data.[17] To assure the consent of both parties, it recommended that a formal written consent by both partners should always be obtained before the commencement of AID treatment. Following the English Law Commission, the Warnock Committee concluded that it should be presumed that the husband had consented to AID unless the contrary was proved, and that the law should be changed to permit the husband to be registered as the father. The philosophy behind these recommendations is clear. So long as there was informed consent by both married partners, the child of AID procedures should be assimilated into the family and treated as a genetic (as well as social) child of the marriage.

In vitro fertilization (IVF) attacks a different problem. A small proportion of infertile women can produce healthy eggs. Although they have a normal uterus, these women have damaged or diseased fallopian tubes which prevent the egg passing from the ovary to the uterus and hence prevent conception. Surgery can help some cases; as to the others, they represent an estimated 5 per cent of infertile couples. As described by the Warnock Report the practice of IVF is simple:

> A ripe human egg is extracted from the ovary, shortly before it would have been released naturally. Next, the egg is mixed with the semen of the husband or partner, so that fertilisation can occur. The fertilised egg, once it has started to divide, is then transferred back to the mother's uterus. In practice the technique for recovery of the eggs, their culture outside the mother's body, and the transfer of the developing embryo to the uterus has to be carried out under very carefully controlled conditions. . . . It was not particularly difficult to fertilise the human egg *in vitro*. The real difficulty related to the implantation of the embryo in the uterus after transfer. A pregnancy achieved in this way must not only survive the normal hazards of implantation of *in vivo* conception, but also the additional problems of IVF and embryo transfer.[18]

Once conception is envisaged *extra utero*, it is possible to think in terms of securing conception with varying relationships to the married couple, depending upon the source, or sources, of the infertility in their relationship. Thus, for reasons of economy and the avoidance of discomfort and risk, the practice has developed of recovering several eggs from women undergoing IVF treatment. Egg donation has been attempted in both the USA and Australia, with at least one recorded live birth in Australia. Some women may produce no eggs but be otherwise capable of carrying, to full term, an embryo secured from a donated egg (perhaps of a sister or another woman undergoing IVF treatment), conception being secured by the introduction of the husband's semen. Developments in the capacity to thaw the human egg (at present experimental) will increase the availability of this technique. The Warnock Committee recommended that egg donation should be accepted, subject to controls.[19]

An alternative technique, necessary in some cases, is the donation of an embryo. One of the sources of concern about this and other procedures associated with the IVF technique derives from the belief that human life begins at the moment of conception. In this view, destruction of the human gametes or their preservation in a frozen state is unacceptable in that it represents an unnatural interference in the right to life of that gamete. Nature is more wasteful in the production of the germ cells than almost any other tissues.[20] Five months before birth, the human female has all the eggs she will ever have – about 7 million. By the time of birth, one or two million eggs remain. The attrition of gametes is even more spectacular among men. If a man with an average sperm count ejaculates, say, 6,000 times in his lifetime, he will produce no fewer than 1,000 million potential fertilizers of an egg. Of these spermatozoa only an infinitesimal fraction is likely to find successful expression in the fertilization of an egg which will ultimately become another individual.[21]

Surrogacy arrangements become more feasible and attractive to infertile couples once it is possible to achieve conception *extra utero* and without the emotional complications that attend normal conception. To date, only theorists have raised the possible use of surrogacy or 'womb leasing' as a means of relieving the busy professional woman of the burden and professional interruption of carrying a child, whilst assuring her the birth of a child genetically related to her and her partner. But some of the opponents of the very notion of surrogacy express concern that this is where the condonation of the procedure will eventually lead. Revulsion at the notion of surrogacy has led to a number of reports, in various countries of the Commonwealth, to urge diverse legal and administration interventions designed to discourage or even prohibit the practice.

Thus, the Warnock Committee recommended that legislation be enacted to render all surrogacy agreements illegal and the contracts unenforceable in the courts.[22] The Committee on the Social, Ethical and Legal Issues arising from *In Vitro* Fertilization in Victoria, Australia (The Waller Committee) has recommended that payments to surrogate mothers should be banned and that surrogacy contracts should be legally unenforceable.[23] A Committee of the Family Law Council of Australia chaired by Justice Austin Asche has also recommended that surrogacy arrangements should be prohibited. A news release by Mr L. K. Bowen, Federal Attorney-General, quoted the Chairman of the Family Law Council of Australia, Justice Fogarty (a judge of the Family Court of Australia) as follows:

The reproductive technology with which the Report [of the Asche Committee] is concerned is not just a medical procedure – and it is therefore essential that the matter be monitored by a national body which is representative of all of the interests vitally involved in these matters and not confined to interests which are solely and largely medical, as is the present situation.[24]

Mr Justice Fogarty said the welfare and interests of the child should be the paramount consideration in control of AID, IVF, embryo transfer and related procedures, and the issues arising from them: 'we are not convinced that this is presently the case,' he said.[25]

Other recommendations in the Asche Committee Report include that the use of known donors of gametes who are related to the recipient couple be not permitted; that counselling be an important and integral part of all infertility and reproductive technology programmes; that information identifying a person's genealogical origins be available to adults over 18 years; that non-identifying information be available prior to the child's reaching 18 years of age; and that commercial exploitation of reproductive technology be investigated.[26]

Finally, the procedure known as gamete intra-fallopian transfer is carried out where a patient has healthy fallopian tubes. The eggs and sperm are inseminated in the fallopian tube under laparoscopic control. This is not a case of laboratory *extra utero* insemination. Where the technique is available, pregnancy rates are reported to be in excess of 30 per cent – that is, about twice as high as the average success rate of current IVF insemination in Australia.[27]

Legal developments

In default of comprehensive legislation, cases are already beginning to come before the courts, the most notable of which so far – the so-called Baby Cotton case – involved surrogacy.[28]

The case was decided by Mr Justice Latey in January 1985.[29] An American couple had approached an agency in the United States to find a surrogate mother to bear the husband's child. It seems that the wife was infertile, but she consented to the procedure and the arrangement. The father came to England in 1984 for the sole purpose of providing seminal fluid for the insemination of the surrogate mother. Conception resulted. The husband and wife travelled to England upon the birth of the child in January 1985. However, the matter caught the attention of the media. Wardship proceedings were commenced in the High Court. In the end, Mr Justice Latey granted care and control of the baby to the husband and wife (described as Mr and Mrs A) and gave leave for the baby to be taken out of the jurisdiction to be brought up in the United States, although the child remained a ward of the English court. The judge stressed that the method used to produce the child, and the commercial aspects involved, raised delicate problems of ethics, morality and social desirability. However, these were not of his concern. The baby having been born, the guiding principle was its best interests.

Such was the public outcry that the British government introduced the Surrogacy Arrangements Bill 1985 following this aspect of the Warnock Committee's recommendations. The Bill proposed the prohibition of both the recruitment of women as surrogate mothers and the negotiation of surrogacy arrangements by agencies acting on a commercial basis. It also prohibited advertising of surrogacy arrangements throughout the UK.[30] Legislation to make it an offence to publish any advertisements or notices likely to induce a person to become a surrogate mother has also been enacted in the Australian State of Victoria.[31] However, this legislation has lately been criticized by the Australian pioneers in IVF on the basis that it has frustrated their research by delaying decisions upon research on embryos created from frozen eggs.[32] The legislation is also open to the criticism that it attacks surrogacy only half-heartedly by addressing itself to the commercial aspects only whilst not actually forbidding voluntary non-commercial arrangements.[33]

Unsatisfactory legislation

Already in Australia, three federal Acts refer to the status of children born as a result of IVF procedures. The Marriage Act 1961 (Aust) s. 92(3) was inserted in 1985. This is a cautionary provision, of local constitutional significance, designed to clarify the intention of the Federal Parliament and to make plain that it has *not* 'covered the field' so as to prevent the valid operation of state and territory law dealing with the status of children born as a result of AI or IVF.

The Family Law Act 1975 (Aust) was amended in 1983 by the insertion of s. 5A. This section deals with the paternity of the children born as a result of AI and IVF for the purpose of determining whether the child is 'a child of the marriage'. However, the determination is limited to 'the purposes of the Act', and it does not deal with the maternity of the child born through IVF. To this extent, there is a lack of uniformity in legislation. Some state jurisdictions provide for the maternity of a child born as a result of IVF using donated ova. This raises the possibility that a person could be the father of a child born through IVF for the purposes of the Family Law Act whilst another person could be deemed the father under state or territory law. This has to be contemplated in cases where there has been an incomplete assimilation of the child born by these procedures as a child of the marriage for *all* purposes.

A similar lack of uniformity exists in Australia under the Australian Citizenship Act 1948 (Aust) which deals with the status of such children 'for the purposes of that Act' using, relevantly, the same language as s. 5A of the Family Law Act 1975.

It is not necessary to consider in depth the intricacies of Australian constitutional law as it affects law governing children of a marriage. It is sufficient to note that there are problems in the enactment of comprehensive federal legislation in Australia. It has been suggested that even the inadequate legislation which has been enacted may be unconstitutional, in part.[34] The problem is that, according to a majority of the High Court of Australia, association with a 'household' has been held insufficient to provide the necessary constitutional *nexus* to a relevant marriage to afford the Australian Federal Parliament legislative power.[35] This adherence to old definitions of 'marriage' at a time when social relationships, sexual attitudes and biological possibilities are changing so rapidly, presents difficulties to federal countries legislating on these topics of family law. They are difficulties which unitary states need not face, but they are particularly acute because of the changing social attitudes and technological possibilities today.

Brave new world?

So far as the status of children born by AI and IVF techniques is concerned, specific provision, unhappily in non-identical language, has been enacted in some of the states of Australia.[36] An Australian Senate Committee report has called attention to the quite unacceptable confusion, inadequacy and disuniformity of Australian law on this subject. The Senate Committee has recommended the basic uniform rule that a consenting married couple entering an IVF programme involving donor gametes should, for all purposes, be the legal parents of any child born as a result.[37] The Committee has recommended that appropriate steps be taken to ensure the classification of the status of children born through all methods of artificial reproduction. As noted by the Committee, those procedures of reproductive technology now include AID; AIH; IVF; IVF with donor sperm; IVF with donor ova; IVF with donor embryo; embryo transfer; IVF with surgical extraction of sperm; surrogate embryo transfer; freezing (cryopreservation) of sperm and the development of sperm banks; cryopreservation of embryos; superovulation of the ovaries; ultrasound recovery of ova; and surrogate motherhood. Research is continuing into the freezing of unfertilized ova, twinning, the development of a substitute womb or uterus, ectogenesis or the growth of an embryo or foetus outside the human body, sex predetermination and embyronic experimentation. It can thus be seen that we are on the brink of still more remarkable developments.

The range of these procedures need only be stated for their

significance to marriage and family law to be seen as a matter of plain concern. According to Professor Max Charlesworth, a thoughtful commentator on bioethical problems in Australia:

> Mind-boggling issues will also arise when eventually human cloning, or asexual reproduction, becomes practicable, since with cloning the very concept of parentage collapses and the whole idea of human individuality and identity becomes quite problematic. In ordinary sexual reproduction male and female cells which each contain only one set of chromosomes are joined at fertilisation to form the embryo which has a double set of chromosomes. Through this combination of genetic material from two different parents the child is uniquely different from either parent. With asexual or clonal reproduction however the child is derived from a single 'parent' and is thus genetically identical to or a carbon-copy of that parent. In cloning the nucleus of an unfertilised human ovum is removed (that is called enucleation) and it is replaced by the nucleus from an adult body cell of the 'parent' (this is called renucleation). The renucleated ovum is then placed in a uterus for gestation and normal development.) What is the relationship between the cloned child and its 'parent'? Genetically they are identical twins since they have the same genetic heritage. And what of the legal legitimacy or illegitimacy of the cloned child? Since cloning does not involve sexual intercourse between male and female partners the standard legal definitions of legitimacy no longer apply.[38]

In tandem with the development of new reproductive techniques, and the increased attention devoted both medically and publicly to reproduction, society is also witnessing a resurgence of interest in sexual practices themselves. Previously the precursor of reproductive capacity for the fertile, sexual behaviour is now infinitely more value-laden. The spread of sexually transmitted disease is, of course, not new, but the identification of AIDS – potentially more universally threatening than other diseases capable of transmission in this way – has altered the public interest in sex and sexuality.

The nature of the disease is such that its implications extend into both natural and artificial reproductive practices. The problems and consequences may differ, but the essential debate remains the same. It is widely reported that those groups most at risk from infection are homosexuals and intravenous drug users. Yet it is clear that drug users may be heterosexual, and that many members of the community regard themselves as bisexual rather than heterosexual. The disease therefore is unlikely to be confined to these groups. Moreover the absence of both foolproof detecting mechanisms and a cure make attempts at guaranteeing freedom from disease spurious and unsound.

The HIV virus and natural reproduction

Unsurprisingly, the impact of the HIV virus in natural reproduction is on reproduction itself. 'Safe sex' currently seems to be taken as sex which involves the use of condoms, not, as was traditionally the case, as a direct means to avoid conception, but rather as a device to avoid the spread of the virus which transmits the disease. Nevertheless, the condom continues to provide a reasonable barrier to conception, as it always has done. If people are to be encouraged to have 'safe sex' then there are clear implications for their effective fertility. Inasmuch as the condom is an effective contraceptive, and if the community is converted to their regular use, not only will the infection presumably spread less rapidly, but one can also assume that accidental pregnancy may also be reduced.

However, when the condom is not used – in situations where the couple decide that conception is desirable, or when monogamy is selected as the optimal lifestyle – a risk remains. It cannot simplistically be assumed that the use of condoms is unnecessary once one sexual partner has been chosen, since that partner may nonetheless be infected. Without knowing previous sexual history, and the sexual history of all previous partners, and without knowing the maximum incubation period of the disease itself, there is no absolute guarantee of safety. Moreover, it is also suggested that infected women run more chance of developing the full-blown AIDS syndrome when they become pregnant, and, of course, infected mothers have infected children.[39] The risks to the community should therefore not be underestimated, even when people are as careful as possible about sexual practices and the selection of partners.

Further problems arise also from the resistance of some religious groups to the use of condoms as representing a threat to the natural process of reproduction.[40] Where they are used as a device to block the spread of the disease, the doctrine of double effect may be used,[41] but it is not yet clear how successful such an argument would be for those with religious objections to their use. Apart from these concerns, of course, the real threat may be to sexual freedoms rather than reproductive practices. This will be particularly true in the case of homosexuals in particular. The hard-won liberalization of attitudes towards homosexuality, at least in some sections of the community, seems to have received a body blow. Sexual preferences may be an irrelevant criterion on which to base access to fundamental freedoms, but it nonetheless remains a relatively prevalent one. The fact that AIDS is commonly transmitted heterosexually in, for example, Africa, has not prevented the media from referring to it as the 'Gay Disease'.

The HIV virus and artificial reproduction

Obviously the effects of infection with the virus do not change whether semen is introduced naturally or artificially. However, the consequential legal and ethical problems may differ. For example, the need for donated semen to circumvent certain types of infertility raises a number of potential difficulties. Although tests can establish whether or not a man is infected at a given time, they cannot guarantee absolute safety. To what extent should routine testing be undertaken? Does it amount to an invasion of the privacy of the would-be donor, or are there more important issues at stake? Should donors routinely be required to identify their sexual preferences? And would any moves to do any or all of these deter people from donating semen in the first place?

These questions must be posed, since any threat to the availability of donated semen could decimate at least part of the infertility programmes currently in operation in many Western countries. The utility of screening for the HIV virus will doubtless be the subject of continuing debate, particularly if its effect is to render nugatory a programme which is seen as providing for the legitimate needs and interests of a reasonably large minority of citizens. To what extent can society enforce disease control on those willing to take the risk?

Furthermore, the institution of routine screening programmes may serve to heighten, or redefine, the professional and legal liability of the staff involved. The involvement of doctors and nurses in current artificial reproductive techniques, and the development of practices which become the norm, mean that deviation from accepted practice could render them liable in negligence.[42] Questions will inevitably also arise as to the extent to which information gleaned as a result of such screening programmes should be maintained in confidence. In addition, what is the legal liability of the physician who screens for antibodies if the test fails to give an accurate result, or if he or she misinterprets the results? Should the doctor have done more to ensure that, for example, the semen donor was not in a high-risk category, at the risk of deterring other would-be donors, and is he or she liable to the mother, the father, or the infant conceived by using this semen?

Conclusions

It is clear that the law both can and may be used as a mechanism for intervention in private sexual and reproductive practices. The development of new techniques, and the awareness of risk, challenge our notions of morality and our laws – including family law. Such legal responses as are produced by judges and legislators, if adequate when propounded, are soon overtaken by events. The hare of science and technology lurches ahead while the tortoise of the law ambles slowly behind. Beyond the significance of the developments outlined in this book are even more fundamental problems. These include the adaptation of notions of human rights to the potentialities of science and technology at the close of the twentieth century, and the question of whether or not laws can be devised which are sensitive to the human problems posed by these developments, and at the same time recognize the arguments against them. They also include the capacity of legal systems and institutions to produce the legal responses with anything like appropriate speed and satisfaction. New institutions are needed to provide these responses in a prompt, coherent and appropriate way; otherwise great injustice will be done, and the law will increasingly be seen to be irrelevant, incompetent or obstructive.

Although family law is typically vulnerable to, and affected by, local, religious and cultural factors, more than most, the approaching challenge is universal. It is also urgent. Unless some international and interdisciplinary machinery is quickly set in place which can identify and draft legislative options, there can be no doubt whatsoever that a cascade of legal problems will present themselves to busy ministers, distracted officials and ill-prepared judges.

This book seeks to tease out, and to flesh out, the nature of some of the challenges presented by rapid advances in medical technology, and to consider the fundamental issues which underlie both the technologies themselves and the human rights which can be appealed to in the continuing debate on matters of life, death and reproduction. Few solutions can be offered, and indeed cultural and other differences may predict the extent to which issues surrounding modern reproduction are locally relevant. However, neither technological nor cultural imperialism should blind humanity to the threats and challenges posed by disease, nor to those stemming from medical or media propaganda. Human rights issues remain of primary significance and the law must be prepared to tackle these matters in a clear, unequivocal and consistent manner if it is to have a significant role to play in responding to and shaping developments. Changes in sexual or reproductive mores should not be advocated lightly without consideration and appreciation of the potential for exploitation and discrimination which they may also contain. Technology may have to learn to wait a little for the law and public opinion to catch up, whilst the law must struggle not to lag too far behind. The time to start work has already passed, and the wide range of topics discussed in this book demonstrates the variety and complexity of the moral, legal and ethical dilemmas which already face us.

Notes

* Views expressed are personal views only.
1 *Mount. Isa Mines Ltd* v *Pusey*, (1970) 125 CLR 383.
2 Ibid, p. 395.
3 Havard, J. D. J., 'The influence of the law on clinical decisions affecting life and death', **23** *Med. Sci. Law* 157, 1983, 164–5.
4 See, for example, Universal Declaration of Human Rights Article 16(3).
5 Law Commission (Great Britain and Ireland), *Reform of the Grounds of Divorce: The Field of Choice* Law Com. no. 6), Cmnd. 3123. 1966.
6 See, for example, Matrimonial Causes Act 1973, s. 1; also *Family Law Act 1975* (Aust) s. 48(1).
7 See Law Commission (England and Wales) *Illegitimacy*, Law Com. no. 118, 1982. Cf. *British Nationality Act* 1981 (UK) s. 50(9). In Australia relevant legislation includes Children (Equality of Status) Act 1976 (NSW); Status of Children Act 1978(QLD); Family Relationship Act 1975 (SA); Status of Children Act 1974 (Tas) and Status of Children Act 1974 (Vic). See also Status of Children Act 1978 (NT).
8 See, for example, De Facto Relationships Act 1984 (NSW). Cf. New South Wales Law Reform Commission, *De Facto Relationships*, LRC 36, 1983.
9 Described in the *Report of the Committee of Inquiry Into Human Fertilisation and Embryology* (Warnock Report) Cmnd. 9314/1984.
10 United Kingdom, Council for Science and Society (UKWP), *Report of a Working Party on Human Procreation: Ethical Aspects of the New Techniques*, Oxford University Press, 1984, p. 13; see also Chapter 2, *infra*.
11 *supra cit.* note 9, p. 25.
12 UKWP, *Report*, 14, op. cit., p. 14.
13 Ibid. p. 15.
14 Id.
15 *supra cit.*, note 9
16 Warnock Report, op. cit., pp. 23–4, para 4. 17.
17 Ibid., pp. 24–5, para 4.21.
18 Ibid., pp. 29–30, para 5.2.
19 Ibid., pp. 37–8, para 6.8; see also Wadlington, W., 'Artificial conception: the challenge for family law' **69** *Virginia Law Review*, 465, 1983.
20 Jansen, R. P. S., 'Sperm and ova as property' **11** *Journal of Medical Ethics*, 123, 1985, 33.
21 Ibid., p. 126.
22 Warnock Report, op. cit., p. 47, para 8.19.
23 Victoria, Committee to Consider the Social, Ethical and Legal Issues arising from In Vitro Fertilization, *Interim Report*, September 1982; *Report on Donor Gametes in IVF*, April, 1983.
24 Australia, Family Law Council, Committee on Reproductive Technology, *Creating Children*, AGPS, 1985; see also the news release for Mr L. K. Bowen (Attorney-General), 69/85, 21 August 1985.
25 Id.
26 Id.

27 This is described by Dr I. Johnston (Melbourne) in Australia Senate Standing Committee on *Constitutional and Legal Affairs, IVF and the Status of Children,* no. 6 1985 (hereafter Senate Report).

28 Subsequently, the story of 'Baby Cotton' was the subject of a book: Cotton, K. and Winn, D., *Baby Cotton: For Love and Money,'* London, Dorling Kindersley, 1985.

29 In 'Re a baby', *The Times,* 15 January 1985.

30 Surrogacy Arrangements Act 1985 (UK).

31 Infertility (Medical Procedures) Act 1984 (Vic).

32 *Sydney Morning Herald,* 31 January 1986.

33 Cf. Kirby, M.D., 'From Hagar to Baby Cotton – surrogacy '85', **25**, *ANZJ Obstetrics and Gynaecology,* 1985, 151.

34 See Jessep, O. and Chisholm, R. 'Children, the constitution and the family court' **8** *UNSWLJ* 152, 1985, 168–9.

35 *Cormick* v. *Salmon* (1984) FLC 91–554, 1984 59 ALJR 151 (HC), *Re Cook and Maxwell, JJ; ex parte C* (1985) FLC 91–619, 1– Fam LR 99.

36 See Senate Report, op. cit., p. 13. Note Artificial Conception Act 1984 (NSW); also Artificial Conception Ordinance 1985 (ACT) and other legislation there mentioned.

37 Senate Report, op. cit., p. 58.

38 Charlesworth, M., 'Biotechnology and bioethics – new ways of life and death', **61** *Current Affairs Bulletin* 4, 1984, p. 7.

39 Recent assessment of the incidence of children born to infected parents has reached as high as 1:61 in New York.

40 At a recent conference on AIDS, the Vatican City representative did not condone the use of condoms.

41 Roughly, this means that an act may be done which has a good outcome, even though it also involves the commission of another act which is otherwise morally wrong.

42 Subject to the tests laid down in the case of *Hunter* v. *Hanley* 1955 SC 200 – namely that if deviation from normal practice is to be negligent it must be shown a) that there is a normal practice; b) that the doctor in question deviated from that practice; and c) that the deviation was such that it would not have been made by a doctor acting with due skill and care.

2   Legal issues in human reproduction*

DOUGLAS CUSINE

Introduction

There has been a great deal of discussion in recent years of what
are often termed modern reproductive techniques. These include
artificial insemination using semen from the husband (AIH), artificial insemination using semen from a donor (AID), *in vitro* fertilization (IVF) egg donation, embryo donation and surrogacy. Something which is not always made clear is that the first recorded AIH
took place in 1799 and the first recorded AID took place in 1866.[1]
These two practices have therefore developed over a long period
of time, and it may be that surrogacy – the arrangement whereby
one woman bears a child for another – is also of some antiquity. In
the Bible, for example, it is reported that Abraham had a child by
his servant because his wife was beyond childbearing age.[2] It is,
however, true that other subjects which come under the heading
of 'modern reproductive techniques' are truly modern. These are
in vitro fertilization, egg donation and embryo donation; but surrogacy is also attracting attention in a way previously unknown.

It is not an exaggeration to say that the legal, ethical and social
implications of these techniques are amongst the most important
issues of this century. They will undoubtedly continue to be
discussed, and rightly so. The purpose of this chapter is to highlight
some of the legal issues which arise and also some of the investigations which have been carried out by various bodies both in the
UK and elsewhere – notably in Australia, Canada and the USA.
Space does not permit comprehensive coverage, but in some of the
reports – for example, those of the Ontario and New South Wales
Law Reform Commissions[3] – reference is made to some of the other
discussions. Sooner or later, every country in which any of these

17

modern methods of reproduction is carried out will have to confront these issues, particularly the legal ones.

The natural starting-point for this discussion is the United Kingdom.

United Kingdom

Undoubtedly, in the UK, the *Report of the Committee of Enquiry into Human Fertilisation and Embryology* (the Warnock Report)[4] is the most important. The Report was published in 1984 and surveyed the whole field, much of which is relatively new. There were other reports at about the same time,[5] but earlier discussions were devoted almost entirely to artificial insemination. Given the extent to which AI has formed the basis of debates in this area, it is worth some consideration at this point.

Artificial insemination

As early as 1943, the subject of artificial insemination was debated in the House of Lords, but the discussion did not exclusively centre on human reproduction.[6] In 1949 a further discussion took place there which was devoted entirely to the legitimacy of children born as the result of artificial insemination.[7] In 1958 the Court of Session in Scotland decided that AID, even if carried out without the husband's consent, did not amount, in law, to adultery.[8] Following upon that decision, an Interdepartmental Committee was set up under the chairmanship of the Earl of Feversham to consider human artificial insemination and it reported in 1960.[9] One of the points which stands out from the report is that AIH and AID were practised on a very small scale both in this country and elsewhere and, because the practice was carried out almost in secret, there was neither accurate data on the number of couples who were presenting themselves for these forms of treatment, nor, more importantly, an accurate record of the number of children who were born as a result.[10]

AID

The Feversham Report made very few recommendations, but one matter which the Committee did discuss – and one upon which it was quite clearly divided – was what should be the status of a child conceived as a result of AID.[11] The problem facing the Committee was the anomalous position of the child. Strictly speaking, if a child is conceived from semen other than that of the husband, it is illegitimate and, in 1960, there were still substantial legal differences between the positions of legitimate and illegitimate children. Although that was (and still is) the legal position of the AID child, it is, of course, in almost every case brought up as the husband's child. Despite this, if its status were known, it would not, in 1960, have had the same succession rights in his estate as would his legitimate child. The majority view was that there should not be any change in the law relating to legitimacy or registration of birth[12] but that the AID child should be entitled to maintenance from the husband.[13] A minority thought that the AID child should be considered legitimate and that the husband should be able to register himself as the father.[14] In each case, the husband had to consent.

Although for approximately twenty years there was no further official consideration of artificial insemination, in 1973 a panel of the British Medical Association under the chairmanship of Sir John Peel recommended that the AID child should be regarded in law as the legitimate child of the husband where the husband had consented.[15] That view was also taken by the members of the Fourth Study Group of the Royal College of Obstetricians and Gynaecologists which published an important book on artificial insemination in 1976.[16]

In 1979 the (English) Law commission undertook an extensive study of the subject of illegitimacy[17] and one of the chapters in their Working Paper and the Final Report was devoted to the legal position of the AID child. In their Report, the Commission made exactly the same recommendation as made by the Peel Report and by the Royal College of Obstetricians and Gynaecologists.[18] Precisely the same recommendation was made by Warnock,[19] but it was not until 1987 that the Family Law Reform Act was introduced into Parliament, section 27 of which provides that a child which is conceived as a result of AID should be recognized in law as being the husband's child, provided the husband consented to the insemination. Much to the surprise of many who have an interest in this area, section 27 has not been extended to Scotland despite representations from bodies including The Law Society of Scotland. The response from the Scottish Office – which defies comprehension – is that Scotland will have to wait until the current proposals regarding the Warnock Report find their way into legislation.[20] It seems to have escaped the Minister's notice that precisely the same argument could be made in relation to legislation for England and Wales.

The above solution has been adopted in about half of the states in the USA[21] and in some other jurisdictions – for example, Canada[22] and Australia[23] – but most of the legislation is not retroactive.[24] In some states, the consent of the husband is presumed. Warnock also recommended this,[25] following the approach of the Law Commission.[26] In New South Wales, the legislation provides that the terms 'husband' and 'wife' include unmarried partners of the opposite sex so that the man will be presumed to be the father of an AID child.[27]

In some of the legislation, the change in the status of the AID child is linked with a provision that the existing legal ties with the donor will be severed when the husband is recognized as the father.[28] This was also recommended by Warnock[29] and the Ontario Law Reform Commission.[30] Severing these legal ties could create a problem in a few cases, although probably a tiny minority. It may be that the donor suffers from a condition which can or will have an adverse effect on the child, but which could not be identified by the screening process carried out by the doctor.[31] If the legal ties with the donor are severed, the child would be denied a possible claim against the donor for fraudulently concealing something which had adversely affected him or her. The Ontario and New South Wales Law Reform Commissions recognized this possibility and recommended a criminal penalty for such donors in the hope that this would be a deterrent.[32]

Until the early 1980s the status of the AID child was the most widely discussed issue in the public arena, but more specialist groups – for example, a CIBA Foundation Symposium,[33] the Peel Report[34] and the RCOG Study Group[35] discussed other issues. The Study Group, for example, examined recruitment, selection and matching of donors, and the selection and counselling of recipients, as well as the ethical and legal problems, such as doctor's liability and confidentiality.

Before going on to consider some of the issues raised by Warnock, it is worth briefly mentioning AIH.

AIH

The practice of AIH raises fewer legal issues than AID. Many of these have been discussed elsewhere by the author, but they cannot be described as major.[36] However, one aspect of the practice which is complex is the use of the husband's semen after his death. Mention was made of this possibility in the House of Lords Debate in 1943[37] and also by the Feversham Committee.[38] For some considerable time it has been possible to freeze human semen for lengthy periods without affecting its potential for fertilization.[39]

Thus, a woman could conceive a child by her husband long after his death. In recent years, there have been a number of women who have been artificially inseminated in this way[40] and, once again, the issue of the child's status arises.[41] Because the marriage has come to an end, the child is illegitimate but because, in the UK, illegitimate children have exactly the same succession rights as legitimate children,[42] a posthumously conceived child has a right to succeed to its father's estate along with any children conceived before death. This could evidently create enormous problems for the administration of the deceased's estate because his widow could continue to conceive children until she reached the menopause. The examples which have received press coverage are those of women who wished to conceive using their husband's semen,[43] but the same problem arises where a woman wishes to use the semen of someone with whom she had been cohabiting. The children would not be the legitimate children of the cohabitee but would nevertheless have succession rights.

It would, of course, be possible to provide by statute that it is a criminal offence for a woman to conceive a child in this way, but this would be unjustifiable, since there is currently in law nothing to prevent a woman conceiving a child by someone else after her husband's death. The real issue is what provision, if any, should be made from the deceased's estate for such children. Warnock recommended that legislation should provide that any child born by AIH which was not *in utero* at the time of its father's death should be disregarded for the purposes of his succession.[44] Apart from the possible difficulty of establishing whether a child was *in utero* or not, such a provision has the attraction that it does not make any change in the present law which permits an estate to be wound up on death, but does take account of children *conceived* before death but *born* posthumously. If legislation was passed to this effect, the courts might allow the traditionally recognized period of gestation to become a little 'elastic' to allow a child to succeed to its father's estate where there was some doubt as to whether it had been conceived before or shortly after his death. In the past the courts have adopted this approach in order to avoid making children illegitimate.[45]

Another possibility is to recognize that very few women would wish to avail themselves of this facility, but to provide that, if they did, any child conceived as a result should be able to succeed to the father's estate, provided it was conceived within a very short time of death – for example, within a year or two. This would, of course, recognize the right of some single women to conceive children and it would therefore be impossible to resist arguments put forward by other single women. The Ontario Law Reform

Commission specifically rejected the Warnock approach and recommended that a posthumously conceived child should be entitled to inheritance rights in respect of any undistributed estate once the child is born or is *en ventre de sa mère*.[46] The New South Wales Law Reform Commission rejected the notion of making this type of 'post-mortem' conception criminal and recommended that the husband should be regarded as the father.[47] Nevertheless, for succession purposes, the child should not succeed to the father's estate unless he had made specific provision in his will.[48]

The most recent consultative paper produced by the British government[49] does not make express reference to AIH after death, but says that legislation would be required to deal with the succession implications of 'storing embryos' where the embryo had not been transferred to the woman upon the father's death.[50]

Until 1978, discussion concentrated on AID, but that year the world saw the birth of the first IVF child (Louise Brown). Her birth was the outcome of thirteen years of collaboration between Doctor (now Professor) Robert Edwards and the late Mr Patrick Steptoe.[51] Since then, IVF has developed considerably and now raises some of the most fundamental and difficult issues.

Obviously, on a number of occasions prior to 1978, Edwards and Steptoe had managed to create embryos under laboratory conditions and had managed to re-implant some of them, but Louise Brown demonstrated that a healthy live birth could result. However, despite the birth, despite the discussion of many of the legal issues which arise from IVF and despite the possibility of freezing and thawing eggs and freezing and thawing embryos, the British government did not see fit to hold any enquiry into these issues until 1982. Some six years on, matters still remain very much at the discussion stage and it is by no means clear what shape resulting legislation will take.[52]

Since 1978 IVF, egg donation, embryo donation, research on human embryos and surrogacy have almost eclipsed artificial insemination in importance. All of these issues and others were discussed by Warnock but, as far as the general public is concerned, most of the Warnock Report has been ignored, and only two topics have been discussed in any depth at all – research on human embryos and surrogacy. It would not be too farfetched to suggest that the general public have little interest in infertility, but it should not be forgotten that IVF, egg donation, embryo donation and surrogacy are still used primarily to overcome infertility. The focus on research on human embryos derives from the fact that IVF has led to the creation of surplus embryos which could be the subject of research, and surrogacy has attracted attention because commercial agencies have become involved in finding women who will bear

children for childless couples. Although, in the following paragraphs, attention will be focused on the legal issues which arise
from these various practices, it should not be forgotten that there
are wider issues, such as the allocation of resources to infertility as
a whole and to the various specific forms of treatment which are
available, which, though important, are nevertheless beyond the
scope of this chapter.[53]

IVF

In vitro fertilization is the fertilization of eggs with semen under
laboratory conditions. In human reproductive medicine, the embryo
so formed may be re-implanted into the woman who produced the
egg in the hope that a pregnancy will occur and a child will be
born.

Those involved in IVF realized at an early stage that, if a number
of eggs could be produced, fertilized and simultaneously re-
implanted, then the chances of a pregnancy resulting were
increased.[54] The optimum figure seems to be three, and the Voluntary Licensing Authority, set up jointly by the Medical Research
Council and the Royal College of Obstetricians and Gynaecologists
has recommended that no more than three eggs should be re-
implanted.[55]

With the use of super-ovulatory drugs, more than three eggs may
be produced by the woman and obviously more than three embryos
may result. The problem of surplus embryos was addressed by the
Warnock Committee and this has given rise to many heated, and
very often unenlightening, debates about 'research on human
embryos'. In the parliamentary debates on the Warnock Report[56]
this subject and surrogacy were almost the only issues on which
members commented. Unfortunately, neither of the debates did
much to increase understanding of this issue.

Research on human embryos

In the author's opinion, the proper starting-point for discussion is
the process of fertilization. Once fertilization has occurred, there is
an embryo, and its existence raises the fundamental issue of its
status or, putting it another way, the protection to which it is
entitled, if any. A number of points should be made clear. If, as
many would argue, the embryo is a human being, or a potential
human being, and hence is entitled to the same protections as other
human beings, then the scientist in whose laboratory the embryo

is produced cannot interfere with it in any way and, more importantly, he or she cannot destroy it or neglect it and thus cause it to die. It must be re-implanted, and given a chance to develop. In many instances, the scientist will be only too happy to do just that, but even if the embryo is not properly formed, or is developing in an abnormal way, it would follow that it has to be re-implanted. In the author's opinion that is, at the very least, irresponsible since the embryo may fail to implant, be spontaneously aborted, or result in a severely defective new-born child. All these unfortunate consequences could be avoided by not re-implanting such an embryo.

The view presented above – that protection begins once fertilization takes place – is a view which is espoused *inter alia* by the Roman Catholic Church,[57] but an eminent Anglican theologian who has examined the philosophical writings in this area has concluded that the protection traditionally given to the embryo varied with its stage of development, and that the notion of protection from the moment of fertilization was introduced as late as the mid-nineteenth century.[58] Furthermore, a distinguished Jesuit has argued persuasively that there is no ethical basis for affording protection from the moment of fertilization.[59]

It is important to realize that the creation of even one embryo raises the issue of the protection to which it is entitled. The Warnock Report suggested absolute protection after day 14;[60] this was also favoured by the British Medical Association, the Royal College of Physicians, the US Ethics Advisory Board and the Victoria Committe and Ontario Law Reform Commission[61] because, until that point, the human embryo is not a unique human being and may develop into twins and, furthermore, what appears to be developing as human embryo may be a hydatidiform mole which is akin to a cancerous growth. The Royal College of Obstetricians and Gynaecologists favours day 17, the point at which early neural development begins,[62] and Steptoe and Edwards suggested day 30, when the brain begins to develop.[63] The Warnock Report states that, once the process of fertilization has begun, 'there is no particular part of the development process that is more important than another'.[64] In that connection, one commentator has asked 'So why not start protection once the process has begun at day one, rather than at day fifteen?'[65] The criticism is apt and, it is submitted, the comment in Warnock was possibly ill-considered given that the views of a number of bodies, including the ones mentioned above, point to the significance of day 14.

These bodies justify their stance either by the above-mentioned ethical arguments or by pointing to the benefits which can be gained from research on human embryos at an earlier stage. Although Warnock and others recommended that research on human embryos should be allowed to continue until day 14, they insisted that the types of research, and the places within which the research could be carried out, should be the subject of approval and scrutiny by a licensing body.[66] Among the benefits to be had from the research is not only increased knowledge of human embryology, but also the possibility of reducing the incidence of genetic and inherited disorders such as Down's syndrome, cystic fibrosis and Duchene's muscular dystrophy.[67]

It is clear that these two views on the status of the human embryo are irreconcilable. That, however, is no justification for not having any statutory provision on this important issue.[68]

It is interesting to observe that many MPs in the debates referred to above were implacably opposed to research on human embryos, but neither in these discussions nor in the Warnock Report is there any definition of the term 'research'. Research can, of course, be no more than observation and, clearly, the scientist who merely observes the development of the human embryo can be said to be carrying out 'research'. Warnock's recommendation that 'No embryo which has been used for research should be transferred to a woman' therefore requires further clarification.[69] The Ontario Law Reform Commission discussed this and recommended that ' . . . an embryo which has been the subject of experimentation that has no direct therapeutic purpose . . . should not be transferred to a woman'.[70] Clearly, any legislation designed to deal with this problem would have to define the circumstances in which an embryo may not be implanted. A number of attempts have been made to regulate embryo research, but all have been unsuccessful. The first attempt was made by Enoch Powell MP who introduced a Private Member's Bill: the Unborn Children (Protection) Bill. The Bill received a great deal of support at its Second Reading,[71] and, at one point, a petition supporting the principle of the Bill had gathered 2 million signatures.[72] The title of the Bill is misleading, in that it uses the term 'unborn children' when in fact its object was to ban research on human embryos and the production of spare embryos. The title was, no doubt, chosen with great care and was adopted by others whose aims were similar, if not identical, to Powell's.[73]

The main object of the Bill was to require the Secretary of State's permission to create an embryo *in vitro*,[74] making this the only form of infertility treatment for which such consent would be required. Furthermore, the Secretary of State's consent was to be given only 'for the purpose of enabling a named woman to bear a child by means of embryo insertion, and not for any other purpose'.[75] It would not have been permissible to create more than one embryo,[76] thus substantially reducing the prospects of a pregnancy. The Bill obviously met with the disapproval of many – and not only doctors – but it could have been circumvented without too much difficulty since it dealt only with embryos, created *in vitro*: it did not deal with embryos created *in vivo* (*in utero*) and extracted by lavage. Somewhat curiously, the Warnock Report recommended that 'embryo donation by lavage should not be used at the present time' because of the risk to the egg donor.[77] However, in the first birth resulting from egg donation, the embryo was recovered by lavage,[78] and it would therefore have been more sensible for Warnock to suggest that lavage should be scrutinized by the licensing authority. In any event, the Unborn Children (Protection) Bill did not cover lavage.

These Bills failed, and it is by no means clear what form, if any, legislation on this issue will take. In December 1986 the Department of Health and Social Security issued a consultative paper entitled *Legislation on Human Infertility Services and Embryo Research*'.[79] Although views were sought on a number of issues, in the section of the Paper on embryo research, the government merely set out the various possible approaches but did not seek any views on which approach was desirable. All it said was that MPs would be given a free vote, an approach which the White Paper *Human Fertilisation and Embryology: A framework for legislation* published in November 1987 has followed.[80]

Storage of embryos

As was noted earlier, the process of IVF may generate surplus embryos which may be the subject of immediate research. However, there are two advantages in storing such embryos. The first is that they could be used if pregnancy does not result from the first implantation. That avoids the woman having to undergo the procedure for egg recovery at a subsequent cycle. The second advantage is that the embryos can be used for research purposes at some later stage. At present, there is no legislation on the storage of semen, the storage of eggs or the storage of embryos, but it is certainly required. This is especially necessary in the light of the recent announcement that a woman gave birth to 'twins' but that the births were 18 months apart because one of her embryos had been frozen.[81] It is not clear whether the law, as it currently stands, would regard the children as twins, but the Warnock Report recommended that the date of birth be regarded as significant for succession purposes.[82]

If a couple have their embryos stored for use in a subsequent cycle, or perhaps with the view to having another child by IVF, it would be important to provide that the embryo was theirs and could not be experimented with. Having said that, however, the couple's rights in the embryo should not be unfettered. Were the couple able to dispose of the embryo as they wished, it could be sold (which most people would find abhorrent), or they could donate it to another infertile couple. Although this, of itself, might seem innocuous, it is easy to see that considerable problems could arise if the infertile couple were related to the couple who produced the embryo. For example (and one would concede immediately that it is an unlikely scenario), a couple might donate their embryo to their infertile daughter. If she bore a child as a result, the gestational and nurturing mother would be the daughter, but the child's biological mother would also be its grandmother and its biological father would also be its grandfather. Warnock recommended that there should not be any right of property in the human embryo.[83]

A more likely scenario is that the couple die as happened in Australia, where the Rios, whose embryos were stored in a Melbourne clinic, died in a plane crash.[84] Not really knowing what to do with them, physicians froze the embryos but a committee which had been set up to consider the social, ethical and legal issues arising from IVF recommended that the embryos be thawed and discarded.[85] However, within a very short time, the Victoria government ordered the embryos to be kept alive,[86] and many American women are reported to have volunteered to have the embryos implanted.[87] The Victoria committee went on to recommend that a couple who agree to the storage of their embryos should be required to decide at that time what should be done in the event of their death. In cases where the couple had not made such a decision, the stored embryos should be removed from storage.[88] The Warnock Report recommended that, where one member of a couple dies, the right to use or dispose of an embryo should pass to the survivor:[89] this was also the approach taken by the Ontario Law Reform Commission,[90] which also recommended that, if both should die, control should pass to the storage authority.[91]

Another potential problem is that the couple's marriage, or other relationship, may dissolve and the couple may not agree on the use or disposal of the embryo. Both the Warnock Committe and the Ontario Law Reform Commission recommended that, in that event, legal control should pass to the storage authority.[92] It is suggested, with respect, that the right to dispose of the embryo should pass to the storage authority only after any maximum period recommended for storage has expired. A couple who initially disagree may subsequently agree, and it would seem inequitable if their subsequent agreement was rendered null because property in the embryo had passed to the storage authority. That was the line taken by the Law Society of Scotland in their comments on the Warnock Report.[93]

It is equally obvious that legislation would have to provide for the regulation of the types of research which could be carried out, the personnel who would be able to carry out the research and the premises within which the research would be conducted. The Warnock Committee recommended the setting up of a licensing authority,[94] the Victoria committee suggested that research should be scrutinized by the Health Commission or by a standing review and advisory body;[95] whereas the Ontario Law Reform Commission felt that some matters should be regulated by statute, others by a licensing body and others left to professional bodies such as colleges of surgeons and physicians.[96] The New South Wales Law Reform Commission recommended the setting up of an advisory committee.[97]

The author's preference is for a statutory licensing body, as recommended by the White Paper,[98] which would be accountable to the Secretary of State but which would be charged with licensing types of resarch, individuals and premises. There are several reasons for this which will be discussed later.

Egg donation

Egg donation is the counterpart of AID and raises the same issues, the principal one being the status of the child. However, there are two other points worth mentioning, the first of which relates to status. A child born as a result of egg donation has a biological mother and a natural mother who are different people. That is also the case in embryo donation and could also arise in surrogacy. In the UK, the law has not as yet had to decide which of them is to be regarded in law as the 'mother' – for example, for the purposes of registration of births and succession. For the purposes of birth registration, it would appear that legislation requires the person who gave birth to the child to register herself as the mother, firstly because the legislation did not then contemplate the possibility of the person who gave birth to the child not being at the same time the biological mother, and secondly because it is competent for anyone else who was present at the birth to register the child.[99]

For the purposes of succession, however, the decision may be that the biological mother is the mother. Although the law in the UK has abandoned the distinction between legitimate and illegitimate children for succession purposes, it would still be necessary to establish parentage in order to succeed to a person's estate under his or her will. In England and Wales (but not in Scotland) a person who has been brought up as a member of the family of the deceased, and for whom no other suitable provision is made, may apply to the court for a payment to be made out of the deceased's estate.[100] This would cover a child born as a result of AID, egg donation or embryo donation.

The Warnock Report recommended that, where a child is born to a woman following donation of another woman's egg, the woman giving birth should, for all purposes, be regarded in law as the mother and that the egg donor should have no rights or obligations in respect of the child,[101] mirroring their recommendations in relation to AID. A similar recommendation is made by the Ontario Law Reform Commission.[102]

In Australia, there is already some legislation on this issue. In Victoria, the Status of Children (Amendment) Act 1984 has an irrebuttable presumption that the woman who actually gives birth to the child is the mother of the child and there is a corresponding irrebuttable presumption that the egg donor is not the mother.[103] The legislation in New South Wales deals only with AID, whilst the legislation in South Australia, Tasmania, Western Australia, the Australian Capital Territory and the Northern Territory follow the pattern of the Victorian legislation.[104] So far as is known, none of the states in the United States has legislation on egg donation but, given the existence in many states of legislation dealing with the AID child, it would be a relatively simple matter to extend it both to egg donation and embryo donation.

The other issue raised by egg donation is the liability of the doctors. This also arises in AID but egg donation gives rise to a further possibility of liability in respect of the doctor because eggs usually have to be recovered by a surgical procedure. The question of liability is dealt with later.

Embryo donation

An egg which is fertilized *in vitro* may be implanted, not in the woman who produced the egg, but in another woman. This is 'embryo donation'. The embryo which is donated, however, may be produced in two ways. The first of these is by *in vitro* fertilization of a donor egg with donor semen and the transfer, or donation, of the resulting embryo into another woman. This was the method used in the first pregnancy from embryo donation.[105] The Warnock Committee approved of this method and recommended that the child born as the result should be regarded in law as the child of the recipient couple and that they should be able to register it as theirs. In addition, the donors should not have any rights in the child.[106] The other method of producing the embryo is to flush it out of the donor's womb. This method, known as 'lavage', was not approved by the Warnock Committee.[107] However, as has been pointed out earlier, the first birth by egg donation resulted from this process.[108]

It may be that the embryo which is to be donated has been stored for some time and the issues discussed under the heading of 'Research on human embryos' are relevant here.

With the exception of New South Wales and Queensland, the legislation in Australia covers the birth of a child from embryo donation.[109] The recommendations of the Ontario Law Reform Commission are to the same effect.[110]

Surrogacy

Surrogacy is an arrangement whereby one woman carries a child for another with the intention that it should be handed over after birth. The examples of surrogacy which have received press coverage so far are of an infertile couple who have commissioned another woman (sometimes married, sometimes not) to carry a child. The resultant child has been conceived as the result of artificial insemination by the husband of the infertile couple. It should not be assumed, however, that that is the only form of surrogacy. In an article in the *Australian Law Journal*, Mason listed possible permutations[111] and the author has produced a similar, but not identical list.[112] The women who have been surrogates thus far have been commissioned by an infertile couple, but it would be possible for a woman to use a surrogate if she felt that a pregnancy would be inconvenient – for example, because it would interfere with her career.

The Warnock Report noted that there is no provision in the UK for surrogacy to be undertaken on the National Health Service and, where it is undertaken, it is usually done by commercial agencies which charge a fee.[113] For whatever reason, surrogacy, like research on human embryos, has been the subject of lengthy discussion.

Surrogacy raises three main issues. The first is what penalty, if any, is to be imposed on those who enter into a surrogacy arrangement; the second is how to deal with a change of mind by the surrogate or by the commissioning couple; and the third is who is to be regarded in law as the mother of the child. As the last issue would only arise if the surrogate had a child as a result of either egg or embryo donation, it is therefore really only the first two issues which arise exclusively in connection with surrogacy.

The Warnock Committee's view was that surrogacy undertaken

for convenience was ethically unacceptable,[114] and the Report recommended that statute should prove that 'all surrogacy arrangements are illegal contracts and therefore unenforceable in the courts'.[115] This was coupled with another recommendation that it should be a criminal offence to create or operate agencies, whether profitmaking or not, if the object of these agencies was to make surrogacy arrangements and, further, that a criminal penalty should be imposed on those who knowingly assist in the establishment of a surrogate pregnancy.[116] The White Paper concluded that ' . . . legislation should not give any encouragement to the practice of surrogacy arranged privately or on a non-commercial basis'.[117]

One of the commercial agencies to which the Warnock proposals apply already had a pregnant surrogate mother at the time of the Report's publication. The child, 'Baby Cotton',[118] was born in January 1985. The local authority, Barnet, was totally unprepared and attempted to have the child taken to a place of safety under the Children and Young Persons Act 1969. This was singularly inappropriate as there was no threat to the child's safety and welfare. However, the child was immediately made a ward of court, presumably by the commissioning parents, and Mr Justice Latey had to decide what to do with her. The surrogate mother intended to hand over the child and, obviously, that was what the commissioning couple wanted, but the crucial and the only issue was what was in the child's best interests. The judge decided in favour of the commissioning couple who were Americans, and gave his judgement on a Friday but did not deliver it in open court until the following Monday, by which time the couple and the child had left the country.[119]

The 'Baby Cotton' case posed problems which the government thought required immediate action. The result is the Surrogacy Arrangements Act 1985. However, surrogacy was by no means new, even at the time the Warnock Committee was set up. There had been press coverage of surrogacy cases in the late 1970s,[120] and one case, in 1978, *A.* v. *C.*,[121], reached the Court of Appeal. It was, in a sense, more important than the 'Baby Cotton' case, because, in *A.* v. *C.*, the surrogate *did* change her mind and it was also a commercial arrangement in that £3,000 was paid to the surrogate. Nevertheless, the government did not choose to act then, nor even after the Warnock Report, rushing through the Surrogacy Arrangements Act only after the 'Baby Cotton' case.

The Act makes it a criminal offence for anyone to take part in any surrogacy arrangement on a commercial basis,[122] a term which is not satisfactorily defined. In addition, it is an offence to advertise or produce information to promote or assist in a surrogacy arrangement.[123] However, neither the proposed surrogate nor the commissioning couple are guilty of an offence even if they advertise their willingness to participate in a surrogacy arrangement.[124] Furthermore, the obstetrician who assists is not subject to a criminal penalty unless he or she participates in the arrangement or otherwise infringes the terms of the Act. Later in 1985, the Surrogacy Arrangements (Amendment) Bill was introduced to cover all surrogacy arrangements – not just those organized on a commercial basis – but did not succeed because of lack of parliamentary time. However, it is possible to make out a case permitting surrogacy in some instances, provided it is properly supervised: this was the approach taken by the Law Society of Scotland in its comment on the Warnock Report and also by the Ontario Law Reform Commission.[125]

The 1985 Act is an ill-considered measure in that it does not deal with some major problems: for example, a situation in which the surrogate or the commissioning couple change their minds. If the surrogate changes her mind, this raises the question of what should happen to any payments which have been made to her, and if the commissioning couple change their minds and refuse to take the child, this raises the issue of whether the surrogate should be compensated for any expenses which she has incurred.

The Warnock Report has been criticized for not making it clear whether their objection to surrogacy was on account of public opinion or because of the possible adverse effects on the child.[126] The 1985 Act is open to similar criticisms in that it fails to deal satisfactorily with what the public seems to find abhorrent – namely, the question of payment. Payments can of course be made to commercial agencies, and in the author's view it is right that no-one should make a profit out of a surrogacy arrangement. Commercial agencies, therefore, should be banned but, in addition to this, surrogacy arrangements should be unenforceable in virtually every respect. This was the approach adopted by the Council for Science and Society.[127]

It is worth mentioning here that some surrogacy arrangements envisage that the commissioning couple will adopt the child. It could be argued that, because the adoption legislation prohibits payments being made for adoption,[128] surrogacy arrangements which involve payments infringe this. In the most recent surrogacy case in the UK, this issue was considered, but Judge Latey, the same judge who dealt with Baby Cotton, decided that there was no contravention of the Adoption Acts because adoption was only contemplated after the baby's birth and that was not struck at by the Acts, but in any event, the court had power under the Acts to authorise some payments.[129]

It is argued here that surrogacy arrangements should be unenforceable in the sense that the surrogate should not be compelled against her will to hand over the child, nor should the commissioning couple be forced to accept it. Although a recent American case, *Baby M*, initially took the view that a surrogacy contract was enforceable,[130] this decision was later reversed.[131] Courts in this country should continue to examine what is in the child's best interests. Furthermore, the commissioning couple should not be able to recover damages for failure on the part of the surrogate to attend antenatal clinics, abstain from smoking and indulging excessively in alcohol, and so on, although some surrogacy agreements in the USA currently contain such clauses.

The 1985 Act deals neither with payments made to the surrogate nor expenses incurred by her. It seems inequitable that a surrogate who has been paid £6,500, which was the amount paid to Mrs Cotton, should be entitled to retain all of it, even if she decides at a fairly early stage not to proceed with the pregnancy. Likewise, it seems inequitable to deny the surrogate the right to recover expenses from the commissioning couple if they decide, even at an early stage, that they do not wish to proceed with the arrangement. The law should therefore provide that any sums paid to the surrogate shall be returnable in the event of her not proceeding with the arrangement subject to the deduction of reasonable expenses incurred by her. Likewise, the commissioning couple should be entitled to recover from the surrogate any reasonable expenses which they might incur in the event of her failing to proceed with the arrangements. In all other respects, however, the arrangement would be unenforceable by the courts.

There seems very little point in imposing a criminal penalty on those who enter into surrogacy arrangements. The most likely result of imposing such a criminal penalty is that surrogacy arrangements would be entered into clandestinely, and surrogates might be deterred from seeking medical assistance with their pregnancy.

So far, this discussion has concentrated on discussing some of the techniques used to alleviate infertility and some of the legal issues which arise. However, attention must now be turned to the involvement of the various relevant people, such as the patients, the children, the doctor, the public, and Parliament; and consideration will be made of what the future might hold.

The involvement of the patients

Many infertile couples desperately want children and some will go to what others would regard as extraordinary lengths to have them. Most of the people who present themselves with infertility problems are couples and, almost always, married couples. Those

involved in the treatment of infertility would probably give preference to married couples and some might perhaps exclude others,
even if they are living in what appears to be a stable union, however
that may be judged. When resources are scarce, it is perhaps right
to favour couples, but others, such as single women and even
lesbians, have indicated a wish to have children.[132] In their support,
they might cite the European Convention on Human Rights and
the Universal Declaration of Human Rights,[133] which undoubtedly
recognize the right of an individual to found a family; but they do
not, and cannot, impose an obligation on anyone to provide the
means of achieving that end.[134] Thus, it seems unlikely that a single
woman or a lesbian couple would be entitled to demand infertility
treatment – for example AID – to enable them to have a child.
Furthermore, although certain 'high-tech' forms of infertility treatment may be available to some, but not to others, that does not
give rise to an actionable right on the part of someone living in a
health area where some or all of these treatments are not
available.[135]

Involvement of the child

The child is obviously the object of the treatment, but is not otherwise directly involved. Nevertheless, anyone providing infertility
treatment should have the interests of any future child in mind.
Thus, it may be appropriate in some cases to refuse treatment if it
is thought that any child might suffer as a result, for example, of
familial violence.

One important issue which arises in connection with children is
whether they should be told, and have a right to be told, about
their natural parentage. This has been discussed in connection with
AID,[136] but the arguments apply equally to children born as a result
of any form of gamete donation.

There is a sound argument that a society ought to pursue the
truth and that birth records, therefore, should disclose only accurate
information.[137] One must, of course, recognize that, at present, the
birth records are not always accurate and, in relation to children
born as a result of gamete donation, it is necessary also to recognize
the interests of the donors. They may not wish their identity to be
revealed and, if there were a risk that this would happen, people
may no longer be willing to act as donors.[138] In addition, an infertile
couple may wish to conceal their infertility from everyone,
including the child. In some circumstances where gamete donation
is undertaken, not to overcome infertility but because of the risk
that some defect will be transmitted to the child – for example,

retinitis pigmentosa or Huntington's chorea – the child will probably be told about his or her natural parentage so that he or she can be assured that any defect from which one of the 'parents' may be suffering will not affect him or her. On the other hand, if the child does not have accurate information about parentage, this might give rise to problems in connection with his or her own health.

Both the Warnock Report and the White Paper favoured the preservation of the donor's anonymity but thought that the child, on reaching the age of 18,[139] should have some basic information about the donor's ethnic origins and genetic health. That reflects the right of adopted children in England and Wales who have access to their original birth certificates on reaching the age of 18. In Scotland, the corresponding age is 17.[140] However, since the child can marry at 16, it could well be argued that this is the appropriate age at which to have access to relevant information.

Involvement of the doctor

The involvement of the doctor may obviously give rise to liability, but under this heading it is also appropriate to consider other matters. The determination of the man's and woman's fertility may involve both a urologist and a gynaecologist. In some clinics where AID is practised, it is the gynaecologist who determines who shall have the treatment; in other clinics, a team will be involved, and the others on the team may include a social worker and a psychologist. Some might question whether a doctor has the necessary training to determine whether or not a couple would be suitable parents. Those who make the decisions on their own would question whether a committee is any better qualified. Others might argue that the state should have a say in deciding who makes suitable parents because they are involved in the adoption process. Others, fearing the advent of 'Big Brother', would discourage the state's further involvement in case it embarked on a 'eugenics' programme. Some might question the entire process of assessing 'fitness for parenting', particularly since it is not apparently applicable where assistance in reproducing is not required.[141]

Where gamete donation is used to avoid the transmission of inheritable defects or research on embryos is carried out for a similar purpose, then the doctor is not the only person involved. However no matter who is involved, two important issues arise – that of the patient's consent, and that of the doctor's legal liability.

Consent

If the patient's consent is not obtained or is obtained by improper means, the doctor commits an assault on the patient.[142] However, this is currently a form of action which is rarely used, and the issue which has grown in significance in recent years is the amount of information which a patient *ought* to be given if a doctor is acting with due professional skill and care.[143] If the doctor fails to give the patient the amount of information which ought to be given, then this is now generally held to amount in law to negligence. The English courts have recently had to consider a number of cases in which it was claimed that the patient was inadequately informed about the risks of particular treatment. The House of Lords held that, provided the doctor follows the practice adopted by a responsible body of doctors in relation of what or what not to tell, he or she will not be negligent.[144] (It is highly unlikely that the Scottish courts would take a different view.) In reaching their decision, the House of Lords rejected the notion of informed consent, which is part of both US and Canadian law, and which emphasizes the patient's right to know what risks are involved in undergoing or foregoing certain treatment.[145]

The doctor's liability

This is too broad a subject to be dealt with in any depth here,[146] but, briefly, the doctor's obligation, like that of the other involved parties, is to exercise reasonable care and skill.[147] It is quite clear that anyone who is attempting artificial conception, whether by AID, *in vitro* fertilization or any of the other processes, does not and cannot guarantee that a pregnancy will result. Likewise, it does not follow that if something goes wrong – for example, the birth of an abnormal child – the parents or the child will automatically be able to claim compensation, although in some circumstances the parents and/or the child may have such a claim.

If parents wish to claim compensation, one obstacle facing them is that the pregnancy will almost certainly have been carefully monitored. Some abnormalities can be discovered during pregnancy and the mother may then be offered an abortion. Should she refuse, it may be argued that the birth of the child is a result of her decision and not of any negligence, and that by refusing an abortion she had contributed in some way by her own negligence. In *Emeh* v. *Kensington, Chelsea and Westminster Area Health Authority*,[148] the Court of Appeal rejected the first argument in a claim arising from a sterilization which had been negligently performed. However, in the context of modern reproductive techniques, doctors may argue that the patient agreed to be monitored as part of the artificial conception programme and that she knew about the possibility of a defect in the child, and hence about the possible need for, or desirability of, an abortion.

So far as the child is concerned, in England and Wales any claim for preconception or prenatal harm would be governed by the Congenital Disabilities (Civil Liability) Act 1976 and, in order to succeed, a child would have to establish that there was an 'occurrence' which '(a) affected either the parent of the child in his or her ability to have a normal, healthy child; or (b) affected the mother during her pregnancy . . . so that the child is born with disabilities which would not otherwise have been present'.[149] Broadly speaking, there are two types of case – one where the parent's reproductive capacity is impaired and the other where the child is damaged after conception. In the context of modern reproductive techniques, a claim is most likely to arise from *in vitro* fertilization, egg donation or embryo donation but, in these cases, the child is damaged in the course of 'conception' and not afterwards. The 1976 Act was passed to meet the problems which arose from the thalidomide cases where foetuses had been damaged as a result of drugs taken by the mother during their pregnancies. It may not therefore meet the problems raised by IVF.

The 1976 Act resulted from the deliberations of the Law Commission.[150] The Scottish Law Commission also considered this matter[151] but did not consider that there was any need for a statute in Scotland, since the common law would be adequate.[152] A claim in Scotland may therefore be less problematic than one in England since the child would require to prove negligence at common law but would not have to meet the requirements of the 1976 Act.

The involvement of the public

One obvious involvement of the public is that they are entitled to take part in any discussions arising from these issues but, more importantly, they are also entitled to be assured that modern reproductive techniques and any concomitant research activities are carried on within the existing legal and ethical framework of our society. It is, of course, extremely difficult to identify any ethical standard to which every member of the public would subscribe and, accordingly, it has to be left to Parliament to provide the necessary guidance.

Involvement of Parliament

Shortly after the publication of the Warnock Report, it was stated that the government would seek to have legislation on the issue before the end of the current parliament.[153] As has been noted already, the government has produced another consultative paper, responses to which were made by the end of June 1987, and a subsequent White Paper which remains to be discussed in depth.

The problem which faces any legislature is to attempt to reconcile two interests which may compete. The scientist (doctor) is involved in increasing understanding of human fertilization and embryology and it would not be going too far to say that he or she has an obligation to pursue research in order to achieve accepted aims. As has been noted above, however, the public also have an interest in ensuring that the research which is carried out is 'approved' in the sense indicated. Parliament must decide how to achieve a balance. The decision it makes may not meet with the approval of doctors: on the other hand, it may not meet with the approval of large sections of the public. It is improbable that any legislation on these issues will meet with the wholehearted approval of all sectors of the community. However, a possible solution for the future is considered in the next section.

The future

It has been assumed above that a government will wish to act in some way to deal with these issues.

The Warnock Committee's proposal, and that of the White Paper,[154] like that of other bodies,[155] is for a licensing authority, and a voluntary one already exists. The White Paper raises a number of important matters, (assuming Parliament decides to create such a body) including its composition and its terms of reference.[156]

Although the Warnock Report did not comment extensively on compositon, there would not only have to be a substantial medical input (using the term broadly), but also representation from other sectors of society, and it is suggested that at least one member of the licensing body should be a lawyer. The body should aim to be as representative of the public as is feasibly possible,[157] although one merely has to look at the number of people who submitted evidence to the Warnock Committee, and the statement in the Report itself that the Committee did not hear from as many people as it had hoped, to realize that not everyone's views can be represented on such a body.[158] A body drawn from as widely-differing perspectives as possible is the best that can be achieved.

The Warnock Report considered a large number of topics many of which it suggested should be kept under review by the proposed licensing body.[159] At the time it did not approve of some techniques, such as lavage, did not exclude it from the proposed review. In keeping matters under review, the licensing body would have to decide in what institutions research will be carried out, by whom and, most importantly, the kinds of activities which are permissible.

It would, of course, be possible to deal with all of these matters in a statute, but such a statute would have the effect of 'freezing' the law at a particular time making it difficult to take account of developments, which have been rapid even since the Warnock Committee reported.

Either of these approaches would be an attempt to balance the scientist's interests with those of the public.

Of course, it would be open to a legislature not to act at all. That, it is submitted, is an abdication of responsibility and would demonstrate an unwillingness to confront issues, albeit difficult ones. Inaction does not help doctors, patients, or potential or existing children. Equally, it helps neither those who support research nor those who do not.

It is submitted that the best approach is to enact legislation clarifying some of the issues – for example, the status of the AID child – but within this to set up a licensing body with full powers of review. The body must be seen to have powers and be prepared to use them to ensure that the licensed activities are carried out for the benefit of patients, children and society.

Notes

* This chapter was completed before the publication of the White Paper in November 1987, but, where possible, the main relevant recommendations have been included.

1 Home. E., *Philosophical Transactions of the Royal Society of London*, vol. 18, pp. 157–78; Hard A. D., 'Artificial impregnation' *Medical World*, 27 1909, 163–5.

2 Genesis, 16.

3 Ontario Law Reform Commission, *Report on Human Artificial Reproduction and Related Matters*, 1985; New South Wales Law Reform Commission, *Artificial Conception: Report 1: Human Artificial Insemination*, 1986.

4 *Report of the Committee of Enquiry into Human Fertilisation and Embryology* (the Warnock Report) Cmnd. 9314, 1984.

5 British Medical Association, 'Working group on in vitro fertilisation', **288** *British Medical Journal*, 25, 1984 (special insert); Medical Research Council, 'Research related to human fertilisation and embryology, **285** *British Medical Journal*, 1480, 1982; Royal College of Obstetricians and Gynaecologists, *Report of Committee on In Vitro Fertilisation and Embryo Replacement or Transfer*, 1983.

6 128 HL. Deb., cols 816–836, 29 July 1943.

7   161 HL. Deb., cols 386–429, 16 March 1949
8   *Maclennan* v. *Maclennan* 1958 SC 105; SLT 12.
9   *Report of the Departmental Committee on Human Artificial Insemination*, Cmnd. 1105, 1960. (Feversham Report)
10 Ibid., para. 22.
11 Ibid., memo. of Dissent, para. 14.
12 Ibid., para. 272.
13 Ibid.
14 Memo. of Dissent, note 11, *supra*.
15 'Report of panel on human artificial insemination', *British Medical Journal* (Supp. 3) vol. 2, 1973 (Peel Report).
16 RCOG Fourth Study Group, *Artificial Insemination: Proceedings of the Fourth College Study Group*, 1976.
17 Law Commission of England and Wales, *Family Law: Illegitimacy*, Working Paper no. 74, 1979; *Family Law: Illegitimacy* Law Com no. 118, 1982.
18 Law Commission, *Illegitimacy*, op. cit., para. 12.24.
19 Warnock Report, op. cit., para. 4.17.
20 Letter from Ian Jardine of the Scottish Office dated 10 February 1987 addressed to The Secretary, Law Reform Committee, The Law Society of Scotland.
21 California Civil Code s. 7005 (West. Supp. 1982); Colorado Rev. Stat. s. 19–6406 (1978). Connecticut Gen. Stat. s. 45–69 f–n (1981); Kansas Stat. Ann 23–128–130 (1968) (Supp 1971); New York Domestic Relations Law s. 73 (1973) (Supp 1974); North Carolina Gen Stat. 49A–1(1971); Oregon Laws 1977 ch. 686; Texas Code Ann 12–03; Virginia Code s. 64.1–7.1; Alaska: Stat: 20: 010 (1975); Florida Stat. S742.11 (West Supp. 1982); Georgia Code Ann. S19–7–21 (1982); Idaho Code S 39–5401–5407 (Supp 1982); Louisiana Civil Code Ann Art 118 (West Supp 1982); Maryland Est. & Trust Code Ann s. 1–206 (1974); Massachusetts Gen Laws Ch. 46 s. 4b (West Supp 82–3); Michigan Comp. Law s. 700–1111(2) (1979); Minnesota Stat s. 257.56 (1980); Montana Code Ann s. 40–6–106 (1981); Nevada Rev. Stat. s. 126.061 (1983); Oklahoma Stat. tit 10 s. 552 (1981); Tennessee Code Ann S.53–446 (Supp 1982); Texas Code Ann 12–03; Washington Rev. Code s. 26,26.050 (1981); Wisconsin Stat. s. 891.40 (1979–80); Wyoming Stat. Ann s. 14–2.103 (1978).
22 Quebec Civil Code, Art. 586; Yukon Territory Children's Act 1984, s. 14.
23 Artificial Conception Act 1984 (NSW); Status of Children (Amendment) Act 1984 (Victoria) Family Relationships Amendment Act 1984 (S. Aus.); Status of Children Amendment Act 1984 (Tasmania): Artificial Conception Act 1985 (W. Aus.); Artificial Conception Ordinance 1985 (Capital Territory); Status of Children Amendment Act 1985 (Northern Territory).
24 In the USA, for example, only in Kansas does the legislation have this effect. The Ontario Law Reform Commission recommended that legislation should be retroactive. Rec. 19(4).
25 Warnock Report, op. cit., para. 4.24.
26 Law Commission, *Illegitimacy*, op. cit., para. 12.
27 Artificial Conception Act 1984 s. 3(1).
28 For example, Florida; Alaska; Kansas; Connecticut.
29 Warnock Report, op. cit., para. 4.22.
30 Ontario Law Reform Commission, op. cit., Recommendation 19(3).
31 On screening etc, see Joyce, D., 'Recruitment, selection and matching of donors' in RCOG Fourth Study Group, *Artificial Insemination*, op. cit.
32 Ontario Law Reform Commission, op. cit., Recommendation 23; NSW Law Reform Commission, op. cit., Recommendation 5.

33 *Law and Ethics of AID and Embryo Transfer*, CIBA Foundation Symposium 17 (new series), Amsterdam, Elsevier, Excerpta Medica; North Holland, 1973.

34 Note 15, *supra*.

35 Note 16, *supra*.

36 Cusine, D. J., *Modern Reproductive Techniques: A Legal Perspective*, Aldershot, Gower, 1988.

37 Lord Brabazon of Tara, col. 823.

38 Feversham Report, op. cit., para. 60.

39 Sherman, J. K., 'Historical synopsis of human semen cyrobanking' in David, G. and Price, W. S. (eds), *Human Artificial Insemination and Semen Preservation*, New York, Plenum Publishing, 1980, p. 95.

40 *The Times*, 11 July 1977; *The Times*, 11 July 1984; *The Times*, 30 July 1985.

41 Cuisine, D. J., 'Artificial insemination using the husband's semen after death' **3** *Journal of Medical Ethics*, 163, 1977; Sappideen, C., 'Life after death' – sperm banks, wills and perpetuities', **53** *Australian Law Journal*, 1979, 311.

42 Law Reform (Parent and Child) (Scotland) Act 1986; Family Law Reform Act 1987.

43 See press coverage in note 40 *supra*.

44 Warnock Report, op. cit., para. 10;09; also para. 10.15 (child born from frozen embryo).

45 *Currie v. Currie* 1950 SC 10 (336 days not ruled out); see also *Preston-Jones* v. *Preston-Jones* 1951 AC 391 (360 days regarded as excessive in the absence of medical evidence).

46 Ontario Law Reform Commission, op. cit., Recommendation 21(2).

47 NSW Law Reform Commission, op. cit., Recommendation 27.

48 Ibid., Recommendation 31.

49 *Legislation on Human Infertility Services and Embryo Research: A Consultation Paper*, Cm. 46/1986.

50 Ibid., para. 35.

51 Edwards, R., and Steptoe, P., *A Matter of Life*, London, Hutchinson, 1980.

52 The consultation paper did not cover all the topics discussed by Warnock. See *Human Fertilisation and Embryology: A Framework for Legislation* Cmd. 259, 1987 (White Paper).

53 For further discussion, see Chapters 7 and 9 infra.

54 Edwards, R., and Steptoe, P., 'Current status of in vitro fertilisation and implantation of human embryos', *Lancet*, vol. 2, 1983.

55 Medical Research Council, *First Report of the Voluntary Licensing Authority for Human In Vitro Fertilisation and Embryology*, 1986.

56 HL Deb. vol. 456, cols 535–593, 31 October 1984; H. C. Deb. vol. 68, cols 528–590, November 28 1984.

57 *In Vitro Fertilisation: Morality and Public Policy*, Catholic Information Services, 1983.

58 Dunstan, G. R., 'The moral status of the human embryo: a tradition recalled' **10** *Journal of Medical Ethics*, 38, 1984.

59 Mahoney, J., *Bioethics and Belief*, London, Sheed & Ward, 1984.

60 Warnock Report, op. cit., para 11.22.

61 British Medical Association, 'Interim Report on human in vitro fertilisation and embryo replacement' *British Medical Journal*, 1984, 286, 1594 Royal College of Physicians *Research Related to Human Fertilisation*, 1982; US Ethics Advisory Board, *Health, Education and Welfare support of Research involving In Vitro Fertilisation and Embryo Transfer*, Victoria Committee, op. cit., para. 3.29; Ontario Law Reform Commission, op. cit., Recommendation 31.

62 RCOG *Report*, note 5, *supra*, para. 13.8.

63 *Guardian*, 16 April 1984.

64   Warnock Report, op. cit., para. 11.19.
65   Lee, S., *Law and Morals: Warnock, Gillick and Beyond*, Oxford University Press, 1986, p. 41.
66   Warnock Report, op. cit., para. 13.3 *et seq.*
67   see letter to *The Times* from Professor Sir M. C. Macnaughton, President of the RCOG, 26 November 1984.
68   Indeed para. 30 of the 1987 Government White Paper, note 52, *supra* proposes legislation, but unusually offers two diametrically opposed proposals for discussion.
69   Warnock Report, op. cit., par 11.22.
70   Ontario Law Reform Commission, op. cit., Recommendation 30.
71   HC Deb. vol. 73, cols 641–702, 15 February 1985.
72   HC Deb vol. 73, col. 684.
73   A second Bill was introduced in the House of Commons on 24 January 1986, and a third on 31 October 1986.
74   The Unborn Children (Protection) Bill, cl. 1(1).
75   Ibid., cl.1(2).
76   Ibid., cl.1(2)
77   Warnock Report, op. cit., para. 7.5.
78   Trounson, A., *et al.*, 'Pregnancy established in an infertile patient after transfer of a donated embryo' *British Medical Journal*, 286, 1983, 835.
79   Department of Health and Social Security *Legislation on Human infertility Services and Embryo research'*, Cmnd. 46, 1986.
80   White Paper, *op. cit.*, para. 80; also notes 52 and 68 *supra*.
81   *The Times*, 24 April 1987.
82   Warnock Report, op. cit., para. 10.14.
83   Ibid., para. 10.11.
84   *New York Times*, 21 June 1984; State of Victoria, Committee to Consider the Social, Ethical and Legal Issues Arising from In Vitro Fertilisation, *Report on the Disposition of Embryos produced by In vitro Fertilisation* August 1984, paras. 2.14, 2.19.
85   Victoria Committee's *Report on the Disposition of Embryos*, op. cit., para. 2.18.
86   *The Times*, 25 October 1984.
87   *The Times*, 25 October 1984.
88   Victoria Committee, *Report on the Disposition of Embryos*, op. cit., paras. 2.17–2.18.
89   Warnock Report, op. cit., para. 10.12.
90   Ontario Law Reform Commission, op. cit., Recommendation 27.
91   Warnock Report, para. 10.12; Ontario Law Reform Commission, op. cit., Recommendation 27.
92   Warnock Report, para. 10.13; Ontario Law Reform Commission, op. cit., Recommendation 27.
93   Law Society of Scotland, op. cit., 1983. Comment on para. 10.12.
94   Warnock Report, op. cit., para. 13.3. *et seq.* The White Paper, note 52, *supra*, recommends the establishment of a statutory licensing authority.
95   Victoria Committee, *Report on the Disposition of Embryos*, op. cit., para. 5.4.
96   Ontario Law Reform Commission, op. cit., Recommendation 67 and vol. 2, pp. 236 *et seq.*
97   NSW Law Reform Commission, op. cit., Chapter 15, paras 1 and 2.
98   See note 94, *supra*.
99   Registration of Births, Deaths and Marriages (Scotland) Act 1965 s. 14; Births and Deaths Registration Act 1953 s. 1.
100 Inheritance (Provisions for Family and Dependents) Act 1975.
101 Warnock Report, op. cit., para. 6.8.

102   Ontario Law Reform Commission, op. cit., Recommendations 20–21.
103   The Status of Children (Amendment) Act 1984 (Victoria), s. 5.
104   Note 23, *supra*. In 1986, legislation was in contemplation in Queensland. It is not known whether it has been enacted as yet.
105   Note 77, *supra*.
106   Warnock Report, op. cit., para. 7.6.
107   Ibid., para. 7.4.
108   Note 77, *supra*.
109   Note 23, *supra*.
110   Ontario Law Reform Commission, op. cit., Recommendations 20–21.
111   Mason, S., 'Abnormal conception, *Australian Law Journal*, 347, 1982.
112   Cusine, op. cit., note 36, *supra* Appendix.
113   Warnock Report, op. cit., para. 8.4.
114   Ibid., para. 8.17.
115   Ibid., para. 8.19.
116   Ibid., para. 8.18.
117   White paper, op. cit., para. 73; the future of surrogacy however, they leave in the hands of the Statutory Licensing Authority (para. 75).
118   Cotton, Kim and Winn, D., *Baby Cotton: For Love and Money*, London, Dorling Kindersley, 1985.
119   'In Re a Baby', *The Times*, 15 January, 1985.
120   For example, *The Sunday Times*, 4 June 1978; *The Times*, 21 June 1978; *The Scotsman*, 9 July 1979.
121   *A.* v. *C.*, 6 *Fam. Law* 170.
122   The Surrogacy Arrangements Act 1985, s. 2.
123   Ibid., s. 3.
124   Ibid., s. 2(2).
125   Law Society of Scotland, 1983, p. 12: Ontario Law Reform Commission, op. cit., Recommendations 34–66. See also Chapter 7, infra.
126   Lee, op. cit., p. 39.
127   Council for Science and Society, *Human Procreation: Ethical Aspects of the New Techniques*, Oxford University Press, 1984.
128   Adoption (Scotland) Act 1978 s. 51; Adoption Act 1976 s. 57.
129   Adoption Application Surrogacy AA 212/86.
130   *The Times*, 2 April 1987.
131   *Guardian*, 4 February 1988.
132   'Lesbian couples: should help extend to AID?', Case Conference (1978) 4, *Journal of Medical Ethics*, 91; Snowden R. and Mitchell G. R., *The Artificial Family*, London, Unwin Paperbacks, 1980, pp. 117–18.
133   Universal Declaration of Human Rights, Art. 16; European Convention art. 12. on Human Rights.
134   McLean, S. A. M., 'The right to reproduce' in Campbell T., Goldberg D., McLean S. and Mullen T. (eds), *Human Rights: From Rhetoric to Reality*, Oxford, Basil Blackwell, 1986, p. 99. In any event it is not entirely clear that the rights guaranteed link marriage and founding a family; see McLean, S. A. M. and Campbell, T. D., 'Sterilisation' in McLean, S. A. M. (ed), *Legal Issues in Medicine*, Aldershot, Gower, 1981.
135   R v. *Secretary of State for Social Services etc., ex parte Hincks and ors.* 18 March 1980.
136   Snowden and Mitchell op. cit., note 128, *supra.* pp. 82–5. See also Chapter 9 *infra*.
137   Triselotis, J., *In Search of Origins: The Experience of Adopted Children*, London, Routledge and Kegan Paul, 1973, *passim*.
138   The consultative paper makes reference to recent experience in Sweden

which suggests that donors would be disinclined to participate if their identities were known, para. 29.

139   Warnock Report, op. cit., para. 4.21; White Paper, op. cit., para. 83.

140   Adoption Act 1976 (Scotland) s. 51; Adoption (Scotland) Act 1978 s. 45.

141   Although recently British courts have been prepared to consider fitness for parenting as an issue – see, for example, *T* v. *T*, *The Times*, 1987.

142   For further discussion, see Chapter 9, in this volume; also Walker, D. M., *The Law of Delict in Scotland* (2nd edn revised), Edinburgh, W. Green and Son, 1981, p. 496; *Sidaway* v. *Board of Governors of Bethlem Royal and the Maudsley Hospital* [1985] 1 All ER 643.

143   *Sidaway, supra cit.* note 138.

144   Ibid., *supra cit.* note 138, *Chatterton* v. *Gerson* [1981] 1 All ER. 257.

145   *Canterbury* v. *Spence* (1972) 464 F 2d 772, US app. DC.; *Reibl* v. *Hughes* (1980) 114 DLR (ed.) 1 (Can Sup. Ct).

146   But see Cameron, J. A., *Medical Negligence*, Edinburgh, The Law Society of Scotland, 1983; Brazier M., *Medicine, Patients and the Law*, Harmondsworth, Penguin, 1987, pp. 55–68.

147   *Hunter* v *Hanley* (1955) SC 200; *Whitehouse* v. *Jordan* [1981] 1 All ER 267.

148   *Emeh* v *Kensington, Chelsea and Westminster Area Health Authority* [1984] 3 All ER 1044.

149   Congenital Disabilities (Civil Liability) Act 1976, s. 1(2).

150   The Law Commission of England and Wales, *Report on Injuries to Unborn Children* Cmnd 5709/1974.

151   The Scottish Law Commission, *Liability for Ante-Natal Injury* Cmnd 5371/1973.

152   *Liability for Ante Natal Injury*, note 151, *supra*, para. 4.

153   *The Times*, 1 February 1985.

154   Warnock Report, op. cit., para. 13.3; White Paper, op. cit. para 11.

155   See notes 94–96, *supra*.

156   See White Paper, note 52, *supra*, paras 13–19.

157   In para. 17, the White Paper indicates that 'The Secretary of State will aim to arrive at a membership with a wide and balanced mix of views and experience . . .'

158   Warnock Report, op. cit., para. 1.7.

159   For example, AID, IVF, egg and embryo donation.

3   Abortion and the law

Ken Mason

Most doctors, when asked what constitutes the law as regards abortion in Great Britain, will reply that it lies in the Abortion Act 1967. This view is incorrect; the law remains as stated in the English and Welsh statute, the Offences Against the Person Act 1861, ss. 58,59 and 60, and as it lies in the common law of Scotland. The definitive law of England and Wales thus reads:

> S. 58. Every woman, being with child, who, with intent to procure her own miscarriage, shall unlawfully administer to herself any poison or other noxious thing, or shall unlawfully use any instrument or other means whatsoever with the like intent and whosoever, with intent to procure the miscarriage of any woman whether she be or be not with child, shall unlawfully administer to her or cause to be taken by her any poison or other noxious thing, or shall unlawfully use any instrument or other means whatsoever that like intent, shall be guilty of an offence.[1]
> S. 59. Whosoever shall unlawfully supply or procure any poison or other noxious thing, or any instrument or thing whatsoever, knowing that the same is intended to be unlawfully used or employed with intent to procure the miscarriage of any woman, whether she be or be not with child, shall be guilty of an offence.[2]

Despite appearances to the contrary, this also approximately states the statute law in those Commonwealth countries whose legislation is based on the English model – the Australian states, of both common law and criminal code jurisdictions, provide typical examples. The 1861 Act runs to Northern Ireland, where the Infant Life (Preservation) Act 1929 is copied in the Criminal Justice Act (NI) 1945, s. 25.

Because of its different derivation, the law of Scotland as to abortion[3] differs in some respects from that of England and Wales, the most important distinction being that, in Scotland, a woman must be demonstrably pregnant before an outsider can be guilty of performing an unlawful abortion.[4] Not only does this difference provide a possible defence for the illegal abortionist but it also markedly simplifies the interpretation of actions taken to prevent implantation of the embryo or to promote displantation at an early stage. It is unsurprising that the Scot, Lord Macaulay, wrote such a provision into the Indian Penal Code 1860; as a result, it is part of the law of the several Commonwealth countries which derive their criminal codes from that of India.[5]

The evolution of abortion law

The provisions of the Abortion Act 1967 render further discussion of the legal skirmishing which preceded its passing somewhat superfluous. Nevertheless, that intermediate activity still provides the framework for the law in many countries which have, as yet, no statutory legislation designed to liberalize abortion. It is, therefore, worth looking at briefly.

A minor legal breakthrough resulted from the Infant Life (Preservation) Act 1929, which applies in England and Wales. This, first, defined a new offence of child destruction – that is, the intentional killing of a child capable of being born alive before it had an existence independent of its mother – and, second, provided that the offence was not committed if the act was done in good faith for the purpose only of preserving the mother's life. The motivation behind the 1929 Act was twofold. It was intended to remove any misunderstanding as to the nature of the previously innominate offence of killing a child during the process of birth – which could be neither illegal abortion nor child murder; second, and, in practice, more importantly, it regularized the operation of craniotomy – the deliberate crushing of the foetal skull when the head was impacted in the mother's pelvis.[6] The 1929 Act also introduced the legal presumption that a foetus which had achieved 28 weeks' gestation was capable of being born alive; it did not imply the converse – that is, that a foetus of less than 28 weeks' gestation was *not* capable of being born alive.

Nevertheless, although the Act was not concerned with abortion as such, it was to have a profound influence in this field – a development which came to a head in the seminal case of *R. v. Bourne*.[7] The essence of the Bourne case is that the surgeon, a man of impeccable standing within his profession, notified the authorities that he intended terminating the pregnancy, resulting from a particularly unpleasant rape, of a 15 year-old girl; he was subsequently charged under the Offences Against the Person Act 1861, s. 58. The judge, however, effectively chose to apply the 1929

Act to any termination performed in good faith by a registered
medical practitioner:

> In my opinion the word 'unlawfully' [in s. 58 of the 1861 Act], is not
> a meaningless word. I think it imports the meaning expressed by the
> proviso in s. 1(1) of the Infant Life (Preservation) Act 1929 and that
> s. 58 of the Offences Against the Person Act 1861 must be read as if
> the words making it an offence to use an instrument with intent to
> procure a miscarriage were qualified by a similar proviso. In this
> case, therefore, my direction to you in law is this – that the burden
> rests on the Crown to satisfy you beyond reasonable doubt that the
> defendant did not procure the miscarriage of the girl in good faith
> for the purpose only of preserving her life.[8]

Later in his summing up, the judge addressed the meaning of
preserving the life of the mother. He said:

> [The law] permits the termination of pregnancy for the purpose of
> preserving the life of the mother.
>   As I have said, I think those words ought to be construed in a
> reasonable sense, and, if the doctor is of opinion . . . that the prob-
> able consequence of the pregnancy will be to make a woman a
> physical or mental wreck, the jury are quite entitled to take the view
> that the doctor . . . is operating for the purpose of preserving the
> life of the mother.[9]

The road to therapeutic abortion, in its widest sense, was thus
opened up and was, later, given a further boost in *R. v. Newton
and Stungo*,[10] in which the concept of the 'life of the woman' was
extended to mean no more than either her life or health.

The practical effect of these judicial statements was to emphasize
the onus on the prosecution to prove the unlawfulness of the
termination or, effectively, to prove a lack of good faith on the part
of the practitioner. The difficulty of so doing is shown in the two
Australian cases – *R. v. Davidson*[11] and *R v. Wald*.[12] The principle of
necessity was invoked in the Davidson case where it was held that,
to establish that the use of an instrument with intent to procure a
miscarriage was unlawful, the prosecution must show either:

> (a) that the accused did not honestly believe on reasonable grounds
> that the act done by him was necessary to preserve the woman from
> a serious danger to her life or her physical or mental health . . .
> which the continuance of the pregnancy would entail; or
> (b) that the accused did not honestly believe on reasonable grounds
> that the act done by him was in the circumstances proportionate to
> the need to preserve the woman from a serious danger to her life or
> her physical or mental health . . . .[13]

An almost identical definition was given by Mr Justice Levine in the Wald case.

As a result, there has been no later prosecution of a doctor for performing a termination of pregnancy in either New South Wales or Victoria, despite the fact that the basic statute law remains similar to the Offences against the Person Act 1861 in both states and the fact that it has not been modified by enabling legislation.[14] The assumption is that the case law has promoted a very liberal attitude to abortion and that further statutory intervention is unnecessary in common law jurisdictions. The probability, but not certainty, is that the Davidson rule would be followed in the Criminal Code States of Queensland, Western Australia and Tasmania; South Australia and the Northern Territory have passed legislation comparable to that which now exists in Great Britain.[15]

The legal and medical professions in the UK coexisted in a state of watchful neutrality following the Bourne decision. There is no doubt that large numbers of therapeutic abortions were performed but these were undertaken, in the main, at specialized centres and by relatively courageous staff.[16] There are, equally, no doubts that unwanted pregnancies were rife during the unsettled war and post-war periods and that many of these were terminated unlawfully and in conditions which were, at times, horrific. The incidence of such operations is unknowable – a typically vague estimate puts it at anything between 10,000 and 100,000 per year.[17] In the circumstances, it is a matter of some surprise, and of significance to the debate, that the largest number of deaths in any one year due to abortion in England and Wales[18] was 185 in 1965. In 1966, the last year before the modern legislation, as a result of this activity, 62 persons were sent for trial by jury under the Offences Against the Person Act, s. 58, 28 of these received sentences of imprisonment.[19]

The Abortion Act 1967

It was against this very unsatisfactory background that the Abortion Act 1967 was passed – although not without considerable opposition from the rank and file of the medical profession. The bare bones of the Act are that it will not be an offence under the law relating to abortion when a pregnancy is terminated by a registered medical practitioner if two medical practitioners are of the opinion, formed in good faith:

(a) that the continuance of the pregnancy would involve risk to the life of the pregnant woman, or of injury to the physical or mental

health of the pregnant woman or any existing children of her family, greater than if the pregnancy were terminated; or
(b) that there is a substantial risk that if the child were born it would suffer from such physical or mental abnormalities as to be seriously handicapped.[20]

Some minor confusion is introduced by the use of the term 'the law relating to abortion' as the Offences Against the Person Act 1861 refers to 'procuring a miscarriage': one has to go back to the Act of 1803[21] to find the two conditions equated, and the word 'abortion' appears only in a marginal note to the Act of 1861. There has been academic discussion as to whether the differentiation was deliberate and whether abortion and miscarriage are to be distinguished in law.[22] The subject is, however, one which is of practical significance only in relation to interceptive and displanting methods of contraception and it will be reverted to later. For the present, it should be noted that, although the decision to terminate a pregnancy must be a *medical* one, the wording of the 1967 Act is so broad that the only effective limitation on the practice of abortion lies in the words 'in good faith'.[23]

The Act, however, incorporates additional features which have considerable significance for medical practitioners. First, a conscience clause (s. 4) is included, which permits a doctor to withdraw from therapeutic abortion in the event that he has, and can prove that he has, a conscientious objection to the procedure.[24] Section 4(2), nevertheless, specifically excludes this appeal to conscience if the treatment is needed to save the life of, or prevent grave permanent injury to, the physical or mental health of a pregnant woman. Moreover, although it is not explicitly stated, a doctor's conscience would not protect him or her against an action for negligence in tort law or delict. It follows that a practitioner who objects to abortion and who is confronted with a potential requirement for termination is under an obligation to refer the case to a colleague who is not so constrained.

Second, s. 5(1) of the Act disallows any contravention of the Infant Life (Presevation) Act 1929. The effect is that a termination of pregnancy is illegal if the foetus is capable of being born alive and this, in itself, raises several questions and poses a number of problems for the clinician. First, although the section places an absolute ban on terminations beyond the 28th week of pregnancy other than for preserving the life of the mother, it defines no comparable lower gestational limit by which to distinguish a legal abortion. Thus, to a very large extent, the practitioner terminating a late pregnancy does not know if he or she is acting within the law until the operation is completed. It cannot be certain in advance whether the foetus is either capable or incapable of being born alive because this is not a scientific fact to be established on the basis of gestational age but, rather, is a biological property of the individual foetus. Moreover, the legality or otherwise of the operation depends very much on how the condition of live birth is interpreted. There is, in fact, no statutory definition of live birth in the UK. A stillbirth is defined as an infant which has neither breathed nor shown any other sign of life after being fully separated from its mother.[25] It is reasonable to suppose that a live birth is the converse of this.[26] But what are 'other signs of life'? If they include a recognizable heartbeat, as Glanville Williams has proposed,[27] then the majority of pregnancies beyond the 18th week of gestation are protected by the 1929 Act and the infants resulting from such terminations must all be regarded as persons who are entitled, certainly, to a birth certificate and, very probably, to a death certificate. This is, plainly, an untenable proposition.

The situation is further confused by the unfortunate drafting of s. 5(1) of the Abortion Act 1967 which refers, parenthetically, to the 1929 Act as 'protecting the life of the viable foetus'. This involves a misinterpretation of that Act, for live birth and viability describe two different states. The latter refers to a capacity for remaining alive, and that capacity is undefinable insofar as it depends not only on the quality of the foetus but also on the quality and determination of its attendants. Medically speaking, 'viability' is a relatively meaningless term of generality.

The problem of the definition of 'being born alive' has, however, been clarified recently in the English Court of Appeal and in the House of Lords. It has now been established that, for the purposes of the Infant Life (Preservation) Act 1929, the phrase 'capable of being born alive' means 'capable of breathing with or without the assistance of a ventilator'[28] – a state which, in existing circumstances, is unlikely to be achieved before the 24th week of gestation. Thus, while the concepts of 'live birth' and 'viability' are still not identical, they are now approximated. The former is the less subjective and therefore the more appropriate reference point to be used in any question relating to maternal or foetal 'rights' within the abortion debate.

The American position

Whilst the majority of abortion laws within the British Commonwealth have evolved through the common law, the position in the USA has been dominated by constitutional law.

Prior to 1973 the various US states had developed statutory regulation of abortion which varied from the very permissive, as in New York, to the comparatively restrictive, as in California. Some states, such as Texas, operated on similar principles to those contained in the English Infant Life (Preservation) Act 1929 but the majority followed much the same line as that developed in the Abortion Act 1967.[29] The abortion issue has been particularly hotly debated in the USA where religious convictions are deeply held and confront an especially active feminist movement. It was, therefore, only a matter of time before the constitutionality of the state legislations was challenged and matters came to a head in the Supreme Court decisions in *Roe* v. *Wade* and *Doe* v. *Bolton*.[30] In essence, the Court held that it was an invasion of a women's constitutional right to privacy to limit her access to abortion by statute. It was further ruled that an appeal to the Court was not available to an individual on the grounds that very permissive state laws were invalid because they deprived unborn children of the right to life.

The Court did, however, consider the foetus in relation to its gestational age. Thus, in summary, it was held that the question of termination of pregnancy was a matter solely between the woman and her medical adviser during the first trimester; the Court could intervene on behalf of the woman during the second trimester – an example of such intervention would be to insist that the termination was carried out in circumstances which put the woman at minimal risk. The Court then turned to the interests of the foetus and concluded that, once viability was established, the state had a compelling interest in the health of the foetus and could intervene on its behalf, subject to the proviso that the continued pregnancy did not constitute a threat to the life or health of the mother. This last phrase was specifically taken to be acceptable, whereas an expression 'to preserve the life of a woman' was rejected as being unconstitutionally vague. Viability was assessed as being achieved somewhere between the 24th and 28th weeks of pregnancy but the Court was careful to insist that this was a medical judgement to be made in individual cases. It was stated that abortion on demand was not an absolute constitutional right, but it is difficult to see how that can affect an American woman's privilege during the first 12 weeks of pregnancy.

The anti-abortion campaign in America has been waged with fervour – and even violence – since 1973 but, nevertheless, the Roe decision has been confirmed as recently as 1986.[31] It has been suggested that, were the UK to form part of the USA, the very liberal Abortion Act 1967 would be declared unconstitutional in that, by concentrating on a medical decision as a prerequisite to consent, it interferes with a woman's 'right to choose'[32] – and this seems very probable in view of the summing up of the US Supreme Court:

> Our cases long have recognized that the Constitution embodies a promise that a certain private sphere of individual liberty will be kept largely beyond the reach of government. That promise extends to women as well as to men. . . . A woman's right to make that choice [to end her pregnancy] freely is fundamental. Any other result, in our view, would protect inadequately a central part of the sphere of liberty that our law guarantees to all.[33]

Nevertheless, it is not without interest that constitutional rights appear to be subject to economic forces. In a decision taken after the Roe case, the Supreme Court held that federal or state medical aid funding need not be made available for a termination unless the pregnancy had resulted from rape or incest or that abortion was indicated in order to preserve the life of the mother.[34]

Abortion of minors

The position of the minor also seems relatively secure in the USA, where a pregnant schoolgirl may elect to have a termination. Her parents have no power of veto although, in the interests of family unity, they are entitled to be informed of the action taken.[35] The position of a girl below the age of 18 but above 16 is quite clear in the UK, consent to medical treatment being governed by the Family Law Reform Act 1969, s. 8(1) or by the common law in Scotland. There are, however, considerable doubts as to the lawfulness of a termination of a pregnancy in a girl below the age of 16 in the absence of parental consent or knowledge.[36] There is nothing in the 1967 Act which circumscribes the age of the pregnant woman but, on the other hand, there is no doubt that an operation performed in such circumstances could constitute an assault.

Yet, in 1985, some 4,000 abortions were performed on residents of England and Wales in this age group and it is difficult to believe that parental consent was obtained in every case. The doctor acting independently might succeed in establishing a legal defence of necessity – the moral advantage of maintaining confidentiality in the doctor–patient relationship outweighing that of adhering strictly to the law. Alternatively, he or she might be protected by the decision in Gillick[37] from which it could be inferred that, having made proper attempts to influence his minor patient to involve her parents and this course having been refused, the doctor could give treatment to a person below the age of 16 years provided that the patient had sufficient maturity to understand the implications – a situation which probably pre-existed in Scotland by virtue of the common law.[38] The doctor would, of course, also have to believe that his or her action was in the best interests of the patient. The Gillick decision was, however, confined to the provision of contraceptives; the degree of maturity required to give 'rational' consent must increase proportionally with the severity of the treatment being considered but, within that proviso, there is no compelling reason why the terms of the Gillick decision should not be extrapolated to surgical procedures, including abortion.

In the only apposite reported British case,[39] the court authorized a termination of pregnancy for a 15 year-old girl against the wishes of her parents who were willing to care for the child. The decision was based on the child's desire for the pregnancy to be terminated and on her capacity for understanding the implications of her choice. Even so, seeking the approval of the court is a very different matter from operating independently: the latter course is probably being taken, but its legality has yet to be tested.

Termination of pregnancy in the mentally handicapped

The compulsory sterilization of a mentally handicapped minor – of age 17 but with a mental age of 6 – which was ordered in 1987[40] caused considerable controversy. One aspect taken into consideration by the Court of Appeal was that any pregnancy which occurred would have to be terminated. Such a circumstance arose in a subsequent case where an abortion was authorized by the court on an adult woman with a mental age of three and a half who was 20 weeks' pregnant.[41] The judgement is unreported – indeed, the case seems to have come to light in an unusual manner; all that is currently known is that the judge made a simple declaration that an abortion would not constitute an unlawful act on the part of the doctor who performed it. The ratio of the decision is, therefore, unlikely to be known. Two possibilities do, however, present themselves. The Mental Health Act 1983, s. 57, together with the Mental Health (Scotland) Act 1984, s. 98, allow for the non-consensual treatment of the mentally handicapped when it is necessary for the patient's welfare – and the statutory controls may be waived in an emergency. However, the provisions of the Act apply only when the patient is compulsorily detained – a matter which is not clear from the short newspaper report – and any treatment must be directed to the reason for the detention. Thus, an abortion ordered under the Acts would have to be justified by reference to the effect of the pregnancy on the woman's mental condition – a ruse which has been described as one which 'would be alarming to most people and clearly not within the contemplation of the legislation'.[42] An alternative interpretation of the judicial decision is that a residual jurisdiction, based on the *parens patriae* principle, may persist in the High Court which could, thus, act for the benefit of any persons who were unable to fend for themselves.[43] But the House of Lords, in *In Re B*, considered that very much fuller argument would be required before a view could be expressed as to the correctness of that submission.[44]

Within a few days, a further case arose – again involving an adult with Down's syndrome.[45] In this instance, the grounds for allowing the operation in the absence of informed consent were that the termination of pregnancy was in the woman's best interests and that there was a substantial risk of the foetus being affected by Down's syndrome. Authority for jurisdiction was based on the Rules of the Supreme Court.[46] Whatever else can be derived from the cases – which are, so far as is known, the first of their kind in the UK – they reinforce the view that the law which regulates the reproductive lives of the mentally handicapped would benefit from a thorough review. This conclusion is reinforced by the subsequent decision in *T. v. T.*[47] which authorized both pregnancy termination and sterilization of a mentally handicapped young woman[48] and in which Mr Justice Wood made a strong plea for clarification of the law.

'Rights' in abortion

The mother's rights

It is apparent that, no matter which jurisdiction is considered, the rights of the mother to terminate her pregnancy are very closely guarded. A woman's constitutional 'right to privacy' in the USA has already been noted. It could, indeed, be argued that this 'right' not to be interfered with is dangerously open-ended – there is, as has been said,[49] not a great deal of difference between being inconvenienced by a foetus and being similarly inconvenienced by an infant. The widely held view that contraception, abortion and neonaticide are all on the same basic moral plane, coupled with the acceptance of 'personhood' – or the capacity for self-expression in one form or another – as the measure of human status, must carry with it a warning that society should look long and hard at the possible consequences before embarking on a policy of abortion on 'the demand' of a pregnant woman.

Yet, a consideration of the Abortion Act 1967 and of its replicas throughout the greater part of the British Commonwealth indicates that this is, in fact, the direction in which statute law is moving us. Of the four 'grounds' for legal termination of pregnancy in Great Britain, virtually no-one would argue against that which concerns saving the life of the mother. But the same cannot be said of the other two grounds in s. 1(1)(a). It is almost impossible to imagine a woman's mental or physical 'health' not being affected in *some* way by pregnancy. The same is true of the mental health of the family: some adverse influence of an additional sibling must almost always be found if it is sought. The doctor has no need to consider esoteric questions, such as the relative safety of abortion and gestation in order to ensure staying within the law, yet a situation has been reached where abortion is routinely available to a woman without having once considered the interests of the foetus.

It might be thought that recognition of the foetal interest – even if only of the negative right to die – might be found in s. 1(1)(b), the 'foetal grounds', but, in fact, this is not so. As long ago as 1958, when the law on termination of pregnancy still rested on the Bourne decision, Havard pointed out that termination for foetal reasons could only be carried out legally because of such adverse effect on the mental and physical health of the mother as is likely to result from the need to care for a defective child.[50] Good evidence that the 1967 Act has not altered this position is to be found in the case of McKay.[51] In this case, a pregnant woman was wrongly informed that neither she nor her child was affected by the rubella virus; in point of fact, the infant was born severely handicapped. A number of actions in negligence were raised including a claim for damages by the infant on the grounds that she was born unwillingly into a life of distress and suffering – a claim which is commonly known as an action for 'wrongful life'.[52]

In dismissing this action, Stephenson LJ said:

> To impose such a duty towards the child [as to take away life by means of abortion] would be to make a further inroad – in addition to that created by the Abortion Act 1967 – into the sanctity of human life which would be contrary to public policy. . . .[53]

a statement which, incidentally, implies a measure of antipathy to abortion on the part of the British judiciary and which also, significantly, indicates that the judge has no difficulty in attributing human life to the foetus. Nevertheless, at the same time, the court recognized that there was no reason why a mother in such circumstances should not be able to claim in respect of the negligent failure to advise her of her right to choose abortion. Clearly, therefore, the mother may destroy her defective foetus if she so wishes; and this

may be for better reasons than the interests of her later convenience
– it has, for example, been suggested that a woman carrying a
defective infant may have a moral obligation of foeticide, save in
unusual circumstances.[54] But the foetus itself is denied the fundamental right to accept or reject an intolerable life – a right which
is, nevertheless, accorded him or her the moment he or she becomes
a neonate.[55]

It is also to be noted that the courts have firmly upheld the
mother's right to *refuse* abortion. In *Emeh*,[56] damages were awarded
in the Court of Appeal for a pregnancy resulting from negligent
sterilization despite the fact that the plaintiff had refused an abortion. 'I cannot think it right', it was said, 'that the court should
ever declare it unreasonable for a woman to decline to have an
abortion in a case where there . . . were [no] medical or psychiatric
grounds for terminating the particular pregnancy.'[57]

The rights of the foetus

Has, then, the foetus *any* say in deciding on his or her survival or
destruction? Certainly, there is a right not to be killed after
achieving a capacity to be born alive – as expressed in the Infant
Life (Preservation) Act 1929 in England – or after reaching viability
– as per *Roe* v. *Wade* in the USA.[58] But this is a very limited protection and one which is consonant with the long-established and
frequently reaffirmed doctrine that the foetus has no rights, save
those related to property, until it is born alive.

To quote from the President of the Family Division:

> The fetus cannot, in English law, in my view, have a right of its own
> at least until it is born and has a separate existence from its mother.
> That permeates the whole of the civil law of this country . . . . and
> is, indeed, the basis of the decisions in those countries where law is
> founded on the common law, that is to say, in America, Canada,
> Australia and, I have no doubt, in others.[59]

The extent of foetal rights in the context of abortion therefore
depends not so much on legal criteria as on a moral base, and this,
in turn, is founded to a large extent on the degree of 'humanhood'
which is attributable to the unborn child. There are two possible
approaches to the solution of this problem. The gradualist theory
sees the foetal and neonatal period of life as being a steady
progression towards complete 'personhood', and concomitant full
autonomy, which starts with conception and is completed some
time in early childhood. The alternative is to regard humanity, and
its associated human rights, as being acquired at a given moment

in development; the extreme view, and that which is adopted by the conservative Roman Catholic Church, is that this moment is to be put at the conception of the zygote. The second approach seems preferable in that it evades the uncertainties and vacillations which are inherent in gradualism. Against this, it can certainly be said that there is no positivist point in development which will satisfy everyone. Possibilities other than conception include birth – which has a solid visual and physiological certainty about it but which denies any rights to the foetus *in utero*; viability or capacity for live birth – each of which, as we have seen, has been accepted by various jurisdictions, but probably without a full consideration of the medical difficulties involved in their definition; quickening – which has the seal of antiquity as a measure of humanity and which once defined the boundary between killing as a capital or lesser offence but which is, otherwise, so subjective an assessment as to be useless for our purpose; and implantation which, at least, records the moment of foetal–maternal unity.[60]

It seems unreal to equate humanity, with its attendant rights, to the conceptus or zygote, first, because countless zygotes are formed but are lost naturally and unmourned and, second, because the early human embryo has had no human contact from which to derive its humanity. Both these objections disappear at implantation and there are other good reasons for accepting implantation of the embryo as the time at which humanity and the right to protection as a human are attained.[61]

An inevitable corollary to this view is that all foetal life is of equal value and that all abortions are to be seen equally as involving the destruction of human life. But this is true only so long as the foetus is considered in isolation. It does not preclude an assessment of the relative value of human lives when a choice has to be made – as, say, between the conflicting interests of the mother and her foetus. Given the need for such a choice, some compromise with the gradualist position becomes inevitable and may be expressed in the proposition that the rights of the potential 'creature in being' *vis à vis* the actual human being must increase as its potential approaches fruition; thus, the relative value of the foetus as compared with that of its mother is minimal when it is only recently implanted but will rise to near equivalence when it is capable of being born alive – or, in *C. v. S.*[62] terms, able to oxygenate its tissues in the absence of a placental connection.

There is, in fact, evidence that such a progression of foetal rights is being increasingly accepted in advanced legal systems. Thus, in only the last decade or so, we have moved from the concept of the foetus being *non persona* to being accepted as a living human entity entitled to recover for injuries sustained *in utero* on attaining a separate existence.[63] At the same time, there has been a move from the use of viability as a measure of accountability to one of simple foetal existence.[64] The readiness to balance the rights of the unborn child against those of its mother has, perhaps, been most noticeable in the USA – and this despite the existence of a very powerful feminist lobby. Thus, in *Roe* v. *Wade*[65] it was held that the state had a compelling interest to intervene in an abortion case on behalf of the foetus which had attained viability, subject only to the over-riding condition of saving the life of the mother. The Supreme Court of Georgia has also taken the remarkable step of ordering a woman to undergo caesarian section in order to protect the life of a viable foetus.[66] The legality of this decision was not challenged because the surgical condition righted itself before the operation was performed; nevertheless, the rights of the foetus had been upheld several years previously to the extent of their contributing to the ordering of enforced transfusion of a pregnant Jehovah's Witness.[67] A suggestion that the court would afford protection to the pre-viable foetus is to be found in *Taft* v. *Taft*.[68] Here, the court not only considered the concept of viability but also distinguished between medical and surgical treatment which might be needed to protect the unborn child. The question as to whether surgical treatment could be ordered on behalf of the viable foetus was left open and judgement was reserved on whether there might be justification for ordering medical treatment in order to protect the pre-viable foetus. 'The State's interest', it was said, 'might, in some circumstances, be sufficiently compelling to justify restriction of a person's constitutional right of privacy.'[69]

Running through the legal decisions is the increasing recognition of the foetus as a patient in its own right and this trend, of course, goes coincidentally with the advance of technology and the growth of facilities for treatment *in utero*. There can be no doubt that this will provide further opportunities for conflict between the mother and her unborn child, although it cannot be overemphasized that the majority of pregnant women, and certainly the majority of those who have carried their infants to a stage allowing for foetal treatment, are happy with their lot and want their babies to survive. An interesting possibility is that of interfoetal conflict in the event of multiple pregnancies;[70] the problem is, indirectly, with us in the form of selective reduction of pregnancy, which is discussed briefly below.

The rights of the father

It is hardly surprising that a father may wish to preserve the life of his child despite the existence of maternal contra-indications – the foetus is genetically half his and a father is entitled to his ambitions for a family. However, genetics alone cannot give the father equal rights with the mother in the matter because the mental and physical effort involved in the production of offspring is so disproportionate between man and woman. Moreover, so long as it is held that abortion is, effectively, only legal insofar as the pregnancy affects the health of the mother, it is clearly wrong that any third party should be able to come between a woman and her medical advisers. One can turn to *Paton* again:

> The great social responsibility [of supervising the Abortion Act] is firmly placed by the law on the shoulders of the medical profession.[71]

As a result, interventionist efforts by fathers have consistently failed. In England, Mr Paton, having failed in the Family Division, took his case to the European Commission on Human Rights and was rejected,[72] it being held that the mother's rights must prevail and must, of necessity, be accepted, she being the person primarily concerned with the pregnancy and its continuation. Similar decisions have been reached in the USA.[73] The matter came to a head rather dramatically in England in 1987 in *C. v. S.*,[74] when all appeal stages were completed in approximately 72 hours. It was held that the father had no *locus standi* to bring proceedings either based on his personal interests or while acting as the next friend of the foetus; this part of the original judgement was not appealed.

The issue in *C. v. S.* was, however, closely tied to the question of the legality of terminating a pregnancy of 18 weeks' gestation which might or might not involve a foetus capable of being born alive. It is to be noted that the European Commissioners in the Paton case were at some pains to emphasize that their case concerned a pre-viable foetus.[75] There is minor doubt, therefore, as to whether a different result might obtain were the foetus to be viable or, possibly, when the grounds for termination were those of foetal abnormality – although, as discussed above, these still relate to the welfare of the *mother*. It seems unlikely, however, that the gestational age would have much effect. The European Convention on Human Rights, Act 2, states that '[E]veryone's right to life shall be protected by law. No one shall be deprived of his life intentionally . . .' and the Commissioners' decision rested largely on their understanding that the word 'everyone' does not include the unborn. In any event, the terms of the Infant Life (Preservation) Act 1929 would surely prevail.

It has been pointed out that, so long as the foetus has no right of action unless it attains a separate existence, it is slightly bizarre to apply that principle to acts which are designed to prevent that very state of affairs: accordingly, it was thought, the Scottish child *in utero* might be able to petition through its tutor – that is, its father – for interdict of any threatened harm.[76] The proposition did, however, always seem extremely doubtful and must now be even more so in the light of the later events.

Other people's rights

So strong are the feelings in the abortion debate that several attempts have been made by outside agencies or persons to represent the foetus threatened by termination. Perhaps the outstanding instance is *Dehlen* v. *Ottowa Civic Hospital*[77] where the application claimed to represent *any* unborn child who was to be subject to abortion. The case failed, first, on the grounds that, since the foetuses themselves had no right of action – by virtue of being unborn – it was not possible for a representative to usurp a greater right on their behalf. Second, it was held that the plaintiff lacked standing to prosecute the claims; the fact that he had no individual rights in law or equity which had been denied or infringed would also certainly bar such an action in the UK. The only instance of a successful application of this sort of which the writer is aware is an unusual one, also Canadian, in which a third party applied successfully to represent a foetus who was already the subject of a restraining action brought by his father.[78] The case, however, appears to have petered out and is unlikely to be of any precendental value. Notwithstanding the decision pending in the Supreme Court of Canada,[79] it is fair to predict that chances of any person not directly connected with the intimate family circle managing to prevent an apparently legal abortion are virtually non-existent within the British Commonwealth.

The status of those who have been described by Glover[80] as being 'susceptible to the side-effects of abortion' are of greater importance – the nurses involved in the operations are pre-eminent among such groups. It is true that the 'conscience clause' (s. 4(1) of the 1967 Act) includes the nurses as persons participating in therapeutic abortion. But, as was pointed out by Lord Denning, this option is seldom taken up[81] – to do so must compromise both training and mobility within the hospital hierarchy and may well lead to adverse appraisal by superiors. The fact that the majority of complaints concerning abuse of the Act come from nurses does suggest that current arrangements are less than ideal; one suspects that this may have contributed to the motivation behind the leading case relating to the nurses' part in the termination of pregnancy.[82]

The major concern of the case, however, referred to the extent and legality of the nurses' involvement in therapeutic abortions in

Great Britain insofar as many techniques for termination now include lengthy infusions which are better supervised by the nurse than by the physician. Thus, the main question to be answered was whether a nurse, in setting up or maintaining the infusion, contravened s. 1(1) of the Act which directs that, for an abortion to be lawful, the pregnancy must be terminated by a registered medical practitioner – and the results as the case proceeded showed the judiciary to be very closely divided on the point. The trial judge took the view that the participation of qualified persons other than registered medical practitioners was legal but, on appeal, the court concluded unanimously that the Act was unambiguous: no matter that the physician inserted the necessary cannula, it was the infusion introduced by the nurse which was causing the termination. It was up to Parliament, not the court, to say if and when the restrictive terms of the Act as it was drafted were to be eroded. The House of Lords, however, in a 3:2 ruling took a more pragmatic attitude in deciding that the words 'termination of pregnancy' in the Act meant 'treatment for the termination of pregnancy', as used in s. 1(3). Thus, doctors were responsible for physical acts whilst the nurses were responsible for those things which are usually done by nurses in a hospital setting. Modern termination of pregnancy is, therefore, a team effort. Those who continue an abortifacient process commit no offence if it has been initiated by, and is under the general control of, a registered medical practitioner.

The courts do, however, take a strict view of the team's composition. Thus, it has been further held that a secretary who types the referral for therapeutic abortion cannot be said to be 'taking part in' the subsequent abortion and is not, therefore, covered by the 'conscience clause'[83] – the mere typing of a letter would not have been a criminal offence even under the pre-1967 law.[84] Whilst this decision is almost one of practical necessity, it is one which is difficult to accept in strict logic. Indeed, Judge Nolan specifically refused to accept positively the proposition that the protection of s. 4(1) was *only* afforded to those having direct clinical responsibility for the patient.

Abortion in practice

It is widely supposed that the demand for abortion is falling off, but this is not a fact – the number, and the rate, of abortions reached an all-time peak in 1985 in both England and Wales and in Scotland (see Figure 3.1). The total number of terminations involving residents of England and Wales in that year was 141,101, giving a rater per 1,000 women of childbearing age of 12.97. The comparable figures for Scotland were 9,838 and 8.8. An interesting feature of the trends is that, despite the relatively fewer abortions in Scotland, the proportionate rate of increase in terminations over the last two decades has been very comparable in the two legal jurisdictions in Great Britain (see Figure 3.2). It may be, however, that the equality is due to no more than similar population age group changes.[85] Attempts to compare the trends with other parts of the English-speaking world would be out of place here although some bare facts merit mention. The total number of abortions performed annually in the USA is known to be appreciably in excess of 1.5 million which gives a rate of approximately 30 per 1,000 women aged 15–44 years. The rate and the trends for Canada, where, until recently, legislative control of abortion has followed the path of authorization through Hospital Committees, would be interesting were they possible to evaluate; any figures would, however, be of doubtful meaning as a large number of Canadian women pass into the USA, and the province of Quebec, which also draws patients from the maritime provinces, has individual legislation. A recent decision in the Supreme Court of Canada has, in fact, declared the existing system to be an unconstitutional invasion of a woman's security.[86] It would therefore seem reasonable to regard Canadian experience to be now of only historical interest were it not for the fact that the Supreme Court will shortly be asked to decide the issue from the point of view of the foetus.[87] Indeed, it would appear that, at the time of writing, there is no definable abortion law in Canada.[88] Excepting Scotland, the lowest current rate of abortion within the British Commonwealth is probably that in New Zealand – 9.3 per 1,000 women of fertile age in 1985.

It is still hard to believe that those who drafted the Abortion Act 1967 – and it is remarkable that an Act of Parliament, which has, to a large extent, set the pattern for the rest of the world, began life as a Private Members' Bill – anticipated the operation being performed on this scale in Great Britain. The public, professional and parliamentary indifference to the wastage of foetal life, which is on a par with the death toll of modern warfare,[89] is, at the least, surprising. There is no suggestion of an illegal interpretation of the grounds for legal termination of pregnancy – indeed, it has been argued above that an illegal abortion in Great Britain, and, accordingly, also in those countries which do not have such theoretically restrictive legislation, is very nearly a contradiction in terms. As a result, it would seem that there has only been one successful prosecution of a doctor under the 1967 Act[90] and this was more for the way in which the operation was performed than for the reason it was undertaken.[91] Yet, despite the benign attitude of the Lane

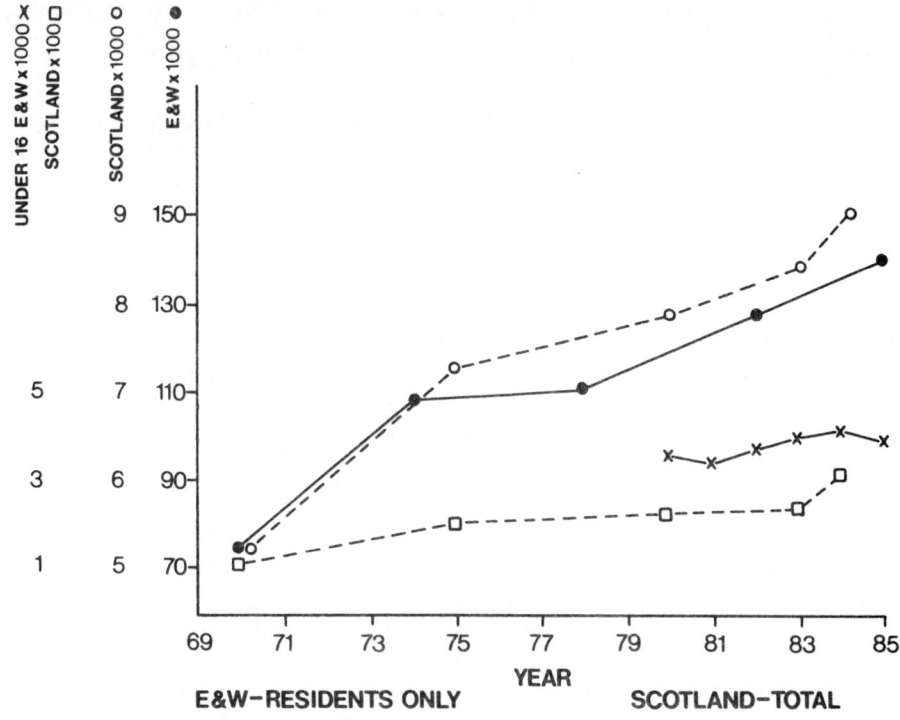

Figure 3.1   Legal abortion in UK

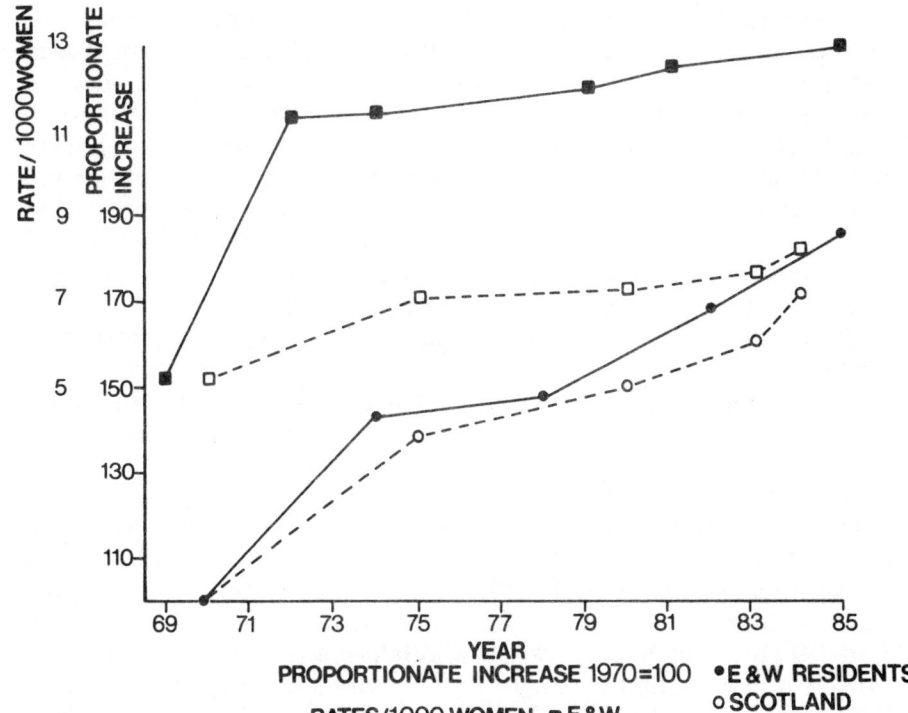

Figure 3.2   Legal abortion in UK

Committee,[92] such a quality of adherence to the law does seem to be statistically improbable; one cannot help feeling that the results derive, in the main, from the near impossibility of defining, or of proving, a lack of 'good faith'.

Is there a good faith?

Only general evidence can be brought forward in an attempt to answer this question; the greater part of any suspicion rests in the large number of foreign women who still come to Great Britain for termination of pregnancy despite the increasingly widespread liberalization of abortion law throughout the world.[93]

By and large, one would expect to find maximum good faith within the National Health Service and the figures in this respect are interesting. The proportion of residents of England and Wales whose terminations were performed under the National Health Service has remained fairly constant at 49–50 per cent between 1974 and 1985. By contrast, the proportion of abortions of non-resident women undertaken by the Service has never exceeded 1 per cent since 1970 – over 99 per cent of such terminations take place in private clinics. The statistics can be analysed in other ways. Aside from emergencies, the statutory grounds for termination which are least likely to invoke dispute as to the qualifying criteria are risk to the life of the mother and the likelihood of foetal abnormality. In 1985, the proportion of these cases dealt with by the National Health Service was 84 per cent and 86 per cent respectively, whereas only 45 per cent of the category most open to an excessively liberal interpretation – damage to the physical or mental health of the mother – were so treated. Moreover, this last category accounted for 96 per cent of terminations on non-residents and for 90 per cent of all those which were performed outside the Service.

There is no denying that such figures provide only circumstantial evidence. Nevertheless, when one adds in such factors that non-residents often enter the country within 24 hours of operation, and may travel in response to advertisement, there is scope for wondering if all abortions conforming to the letter of the law are, at the same time, performed according to its spirit.

But even this is beyond positive demonstration. Reported decisions of the General Medical Council – a function of which is to investigate 'serious professional misconduct' rather than criminal guilt or innocence – as to abortion since 1967 are very hard to find. A study of the Council's annual reports since 1980 reveals no relevant recorded cases. In one previous instance, a clinic had advertised its abortion facilities but the erasure from the medical register of a doctor associated with that clinic was overturned on appeal to the Privy Council.[94] A second case resulted in suspension from the register for 12 months but was reported largely as a matter of industrial law.[95] Thus, there seems no likelihood of any change designed to strengthen the law on this account and, indeed, the British Medical Association has consistently resisted any such alterations.[96]

The under-age abortion

The consensual problems attached to the abortion of minors have been discussed above. In practice, the annual rate of abortions in England and Wales is currently 5.4 per 1,000 girls under the age of 16. It will be seen in figure 3.2 (page 63) that there has been no dramatic escalation in recent years and, in fact, the proportionate increase in the number of abortions in this age group lags far behind the overall increase both in England and Wales and in Scotland.

The number of abortions is not, however, the only measure of schoolgirl sexuality. A review of the statistics – which can only result in an estimate insofar as the age of young mothers at the time of conception cannot be accurately known – suggests that as many pregnancies initiated by intercourse with girls under the age of 16 went to full term as were aborted. That is, in 1985, over 9,000 schoolgirls became pregnant. No matter what its ending, pregnancy at this age must have a striking effect on the physical and mental health of the girls concerned. Given the persistence of the current climate as to sexual mores, there is clearly a case to be made out that the provision of contraception is a preferred option.

Foetal grounds for abortion

The foetal grounds for abortion are singled out for consideration because they form a rather different conceptual category from the others and because they have considerable practical importance in respect of the operation of the law in the later stages of pregnancy.

Termination of pregnancy for 'eugenic' reasons arouses mixed feelings. Many would see these grounds as being those which are most acceptable morally, second only to the saving of the mother's life. Others reject them as an example of the law discriminating against handicapped children and turning them, as a group, into a potentially disposable commodity.[97] It is arguable that the latter viewpoint is valid only so long as the 'foetal grounds' are, in reality, disguised 'maternal grounds'; the point will, however, be reverted to in the conclusions to this chapter.

Terminations on foetal grounds tend to result in late abortions. Thus, whilst less than 2 per cent of all abortions on residents of

England and Wales in 1985 were performed for foetal reasons, the proportion was 17 per cent when terminations after 20 weeks' gestation were considered alone. This latter figure has been rising steadily due, it is supposed, to the increasing number of antenatal investigations which are being made available. Whilst their number should begin to fall with the introduction of modern diagnostic techniques – for example, chorionic villus sampling – 'foetal' terminations contribute significantly to the debate surrounding terminations and viability. Their particular problem can be regarded as part of the dilemma of the living abortus.

The living abortus

Viability, as has already been discussed, is a diffuse concept which depends, *inter alia*, on the perinatal medical facilities available. Given ideal facilities, the one-year survival rate of very premature infants increases from 7 per cent at 23 weeks' to 75 per cent at 28 weeks' gestation.[98] There is, therefore, a fair chance that a late abortion can result in an abortus which is, at least, born alive. Such an event carries with it serious ethical, social and legal problems. The infant who is born alive is entitled to a birth certificate irrespective of the reason for its live birth.[99] Equally, a being born alive is fully protected by the law; a doctor who deliberatley kills an infant stands liable to be charged with murder and, if he or she allows it to die by neglect, may be guilty of either murder or manslaughter depending upon the degree of the duty of care which may be attributed to him or her. On the other hand, he or she has effectively contracted with a woman to relieve her of her pregnancy, and it can only be with great social difficulty that he or she can simply apologise to her for the fact that her baby is now alive in the intensive care unit.

The obstetrician also lacks guidance from the law. Much must depend upon the definition of abortion. Williams says that, for legal purposes, abortion means foeticide: the *intentional* destruction of the foetus in the womb, or any untimely delivery brought about with intent to cause the death of the foetus.[100] Whilst it is presumptuous to dispute with such an authority, it is difficult to see how this derives either from the Offences Against the Person Act 1861 – which refers to procuring a miscarriage – or from the Abortion Act 1967 – which concerns the termination of pregnancy. Neither address the question of foeticide directly – all that can be said is that foeticide is an inevitable coincident when the operation is carried out early in pregnancy. By contrast, the Infant Life (Preservation) Act 1929 – together with all legislation which dictates a maximum foetal age for legal abortion – specifically proscribes late foeticide by defining the offence of child destruction. The doctor performing a late abortion is therefore in a well-nigh impossible situation: in so doing, he or she *may* be guilty of child destruction, or, indeed, of attempted child destruction,[101] but this cannot be known for certain until after the event.

There is authoritative backing for this analysis from the Lane Committee[102] who, admittedly a decade ago, said:

> It is unlawful for termination of pregnancy to be carried out by a method which destroys a foetus capable of being born alive, even if its chances of survival are slight or non-existent. . . . If an alive and apparently viable foetus emerges from the termination there is a statutory duty to try and keep it alive. . . . Further, if after delivery a foetus shows signs of life, an offence is committed if its birth and death are not registered or if it is incinerated other than in a crematorium.[103]

Somerville, writing from Canada,[104] thought that a physician not only had no right to kill a foetus deliberately but that he or she was under an obligation to preserve the life of the abortus if this could be done. Morally, this must be so, but decision-making lies in an area in which there is no legal direction; instead, doctors have to take their chance with the law as it stands, and the outcomes may be capricious.

Two interesting cases have been reported from the USA. In the first of these,[105] a doctor who performed an abortion by hysterectomy, and who appeared to allow the foetus to die deliberately, was found guilty of manslaughter. The decision was, however, reversed on appeal, it being considered that there was insufficient evidence to indicate that the doctor's conduct was reckless or that the foetus was 'born live'. The case of Dr Waddill[106] was even more turbulent. Here, the physician ordered 'oxygen only' for a 26 week-old foetus which had survived a saline infusion abortion. He was charged with murder following its death but the jury divided 7:5 in favour of acquittal. A retrial was ordered and this, again, resulted in a 'hung jury'; it was only then that the trial judge dismissed all criminal charges against him.

Comparable English cases have generally been considered at the level of the coroner's court and, accordingly, provide no legal precedents. So far as is known, only one coroner's verdict has ascribed death to want of attention at birth[107] and, in this case, no further legal action was taken. The nearest approach to a definitive trial arose in *R. v. Hamilton*.[108] Dr Hamilton allegedly abandoned an abortus which transpired, unexpectedly, to be of 30 weeks' gestation and which survived the experience. The doctor was charged with attempted murder but the magistrates took the unprecedented view that there was no case to answer even though the case was instigated by the Director of Public Prosecutions; the matter was therefore not put to a jury.

The evidence is, then, that the courts are reluctant to put the matter to the test and that, when forced to do so, will use such devices as are available to evade the issues. One unfortunate practical consideration is that, whereas it is virtually impossible to disguise the occurrence of a live birth, the production of a dead abortus provokes no comment. In cases of doubt, therefore, obstetricians tend to elect a technique which will ensure the latter end result and, sometimes, this may be to the detriment of the mother – for example, in the choice of a saline rather than a safer prostaglandin infusion. The subject of the living abortus does seem to be one which merits urgent legislative attention – yet even the House of Lords can apply parliamentary ruses to stultify discussion.[109] Whether or not the same fate will befall the Abortion (Amendment) Bill 1987, which is currently before the House of Commons, remains to be seen. This particular Bill seeks to reduce the gestational age beyond which an abortion will not be legal to 18 weeks. Whilst such a rule would undoubtedly solve the problem of the living abortus, it is far from certain that it would operate entirely in the interests of the foetus; the implications are considered briefly in later paragraphs.

The unimplanted embryo

At the other extreme of the gestational scale, the problem of the disposal of the unimplanted embryo raises issues which are of considerable academic interest but which, at the same time, are unlikely to give rise to such dramatic practical difficulties.

The problem relates to treatment designed either to prevent implantation of the fertilized ovum (interceptive measures) or to dislodge the zygote which was recently implanted (displantation). Specifically, the question is: do these methods – for example, the use of intra-uterine devices or of the so-called 'morning after pill' – constitute contraception or abortion? If they are the latter, then they cannot, strictly speaking, be legal in that, firstly, the procedure is unlikely to have been certified by two registered medical practitioners and, more fundamentally, because the practices are adopted only when the fact of pregnancy is in doubt – and the 1967 Act refers to termination of pregnancy, not of doubtful pregnancy.

Thus, the nub of the question lies further back in the Offences

Against the Person Act 1861, ss. 58 and 59: does the use of, or the fitting of, a coil or the taking or supplying of an interceptive pill constitute the procurement of a miscarriage? Although it could possibly be so, it is very improbable that the woman herself would be guilty of any offence because she clearly would not know that she was pregnant. Similarly, the Scottish doctor would be innocent because it is necessary in every case in Scotland to prove the fact of pregnancy before a recognizable offence is committed,[110] and it is also difficult to see how he or she could be guilty of an attempt if there was uncertainty as to pregnancy.[111] The English practitioner could, however, be at risk from the 1861 Act under both s. 58 and s. 59 – that is, by administering or supplying any poison or noxious thing knowing that the *intention* is to procure a miscarriage, irrespective of the fact of pregnancy. Two questions then call to be answered: first, are abortion and miscarriage synonymous and, second, can one procure the miscarriage of an embryo which is not yet implanted?

The legal answer to the first is unresolved. A good case can be made out that they have the same meaning;[112] and the wording of the Abortion Act 1967, s. 6 – 'the law relating to abortion means sections 58 and 59 of the Offences Against the Person Act 1861' – seems good evidence of the legislators' intentions. Williams, however, believed that the term 'abortion' was deliberately dropped from the 1861 Act in order to distinguish clearly a miscarriage which, he said, involves a foetus of relatively late gestational development.[113] It is, perhaps, easier to address the second question and, here, the view that a miscarriage is impossible in the absence of carriage must surely prevail. Substances lying in the lumen of body passages which open to the exterior are, physiologically speaking, external to the body; at that point, they are doing no more than passing through. It is true that the zygote may become caught up and implanted, but it is not until then that it can be said to be being 'carried'.

There is very strongly persuasive evidence that this interpretation is correct. Thus, the Attorney-General, in refusing to prosecute those using post-coital interceptive drugs, said: 'It is clear that, used in its ordinary sense, the word "miscarriage" is not apt to describe a failure to implant, whether spontaneous or not.'[114] Nonetheless, the current advice of the Department of Health and Social Security is that, to ensure their immunity, doctors should only use post-coital methods within 72 hours of sexual intercourse: this is a very cautious approach since implantation is unlikely to occur for some 8–10 days.

This advice leads to consideration of displanting methods such as menstrual extraction or the fitting of a coil with the deliberate intention of dislodging an already implanted embryo. The scenario is now completely changed and it is difficult to see how such treatments can be legal unless they are undertaken within the terms of the Abortion Act 1967 – the fact that the foetus is of the order of only two weeks old is of no concern. Even then, the law as it stands may be contravened unless the Act is qualified along the lines, 'reference to termination of pregnancy includes acts done with intent to terminate pregnancy if such exists', as was recommended by the Lane Committee.[115]

The suggestion made above that these considerations may be of more theoretical than practical importance stems from the conviction that the law would not expose itself to scorn by, say, prosecuting a doctor who fitted an intra-uterine device as a means of contraception. If doing so does cause 'abortion', then it must be that form of abortion which gives least offence and which provokes least general side-effects. The significance of the argument has, in practice, been shifted into the field of *in vitro* fertilization and embryocide.[116]

Selective reduction of pregnancy

Mention of *in vitro* fertilization brings to mind a further instance of the uncertainties in the law which arise as medical technology advances. Occasional instances of undesirably large multiple pregnancies occur whether infertility is being treated by ovarian stimulants or childlessness by embryo transfer. The problem arises as to whether it is either legally or morally acceptable to reduce the number of implantations by selective foeticide or abortion.[117] The legal arguments would seem, again, to turn on some delicate semantics. Thus, whether or not reduction of pregnancy contravenes the Offences Against the Person Act 1861 or the Abortion Act 1967 depends, once more, on the interpretation of 'procuring a miscarriage' and also on the meaning of 'termination of pregnancy'. Put simply, does pregnancy relate to a specific relationship between a foetus and its mother or is it the state of being pregnant? Even if the former definition is correct, it is still not certain whether foeticide *per se* is a recognized crime[118] – perhaps the Scottish legal system would be able to address this question more easily than would the English. Second, it might be asked whether foetuses *in utero* are 'existing children of the family'. If so, selective reduction may well be legal in that the termination of *some* lives would certainly reduce the risk to the health of the others, but the argument then becomes circular in that it forces the question 'is it legal to kill existing members of the family?'. The best pointer to the law may well lie in the fact that, although selective reduction is practised openly,[119] there have been no prosecutions.

In the moral ambience, there can be little doubt that taking some lives in order to save others is generally repugnant;[120] moreover, the selection process is open to abuse. On the other hand, it is very difficult to justify the severe mental trauma and the economic waste involved in preserving large numbers of foetuses in the near-certainty that they will all die as neonates. Perhaps the best answer – albeit not perfect in terms of clinical judgement – is to limit the chances of extreme multiple pregnancies, say, by limiting the number of embryos inserted at any one time;[121] it may be the General Medical Council, rather than the criminal court, which has the last word on the subject.

What is wrong with the abortion laws?

The unarguable aspect of abortion law is that, no matter what form it takes, it cannot please everyone. Attitudes are polarized. On the one hand, there are those who pray for the death of a Supreme Court judge so that the majority in the court who support what is often called the 'woman's right to choose' can be disrupted. On the other, it has been said[122] that the 'pro-choice' movement, in defining the issue as one of absolute rights, has never made room in its public stance for consideration of the foetus. Legal abortion has been with us for 20 years and is here to stay; but it seems self-evident that no-one can be happy with a situation which, at its extreme, leads to personal violence and to crimes against property. A further difficulty is that politicians, on both sides of the Atlantic, have injected party politics into what many would regard as a matter of personal conscience. The task of those who seek a middle way is thus made that much harder. Nevertheless, it is worth reiterating a personal view.

There would seem to be three main criticisms to be made of abortion law as exemplified by the British Act of 1967. Firstly, it is deceptive; second, it pays little attention to the changes in values which arise during the course of gestation; and third, the over-whelming accent on maternal interests denies the foetus the basic rights which it would be accorded, virtually without question, as a neonate.

The element of deception lies in the lip-service paid to the concept of medical indications for termination of pregnancy. The great majority of currently trained doctors believe, albeit wrongly, that a woman has a right to abortion, and act accordingly. On the other hand, the law everywhere gives rights to the foetus which are almost on a par with those of the mother once it is capable of being born alive. How this is defined differs from one jurisdiction to another but, in general, the *C. v. S.* test of ability to survive without a placental connection seems a reasonable compromise – and most authorities would place that point as being around 24 weeks' gestation within the typical perinatal hospital ambience.

Taking these two conditions together, it is possible to arrive at something of a three-tier attitude to abortion.[123] Although it may be bowing to the wind, it is nevertheless reasonable, and honest, to admit abortion at the request of the mother up to, say, the mid-point between negligible and maximum foetal rights – that is, between the pre-implantation embryo and the foetus capable of being born alive, or up to the 12th week of gestation. This would, in fact, do no more than bring Britain into line with such diverse social systems as the USA and the Eastern European communist bloc. Between 12 and 24 weeks, however, the maturing foetus has maturing rights which should, at the very least, exceed those of the mother to personal convenience. The Abortion (Amendment) Bill 1979 proposed an alteration to the overall grounds for legal abortion which would require a *grave* risk to the health of the mother – a motion which was doomed to failure from the outset. Such a limitation might, however, be acceptable – and be seen to be just both to the foetus and to the mother – if it were confined to terminations in the second trimester.

The need for legislation to protect both the foetus and the physician when abortions are performed at or around the 24th week of gestation has already been emphasized. It is suggested that terminations likely to result in a living abortus should be undertaken with a view to preserving that life when the opportunity arises.

This is, however, not such a simple proposition as might appear. Statutes including such a provision have, for example, been declared unconstitutional in the USA.[124] The general reason for this has been that the possibility of criminal proceedings could have a chilling effect on the willingness of physicians to perform abortions near the point of viability and that this would encroach upon the woman's rights; but, in Great Britain, it is implicit that the 1967 Act provides no legal backing for such 'rights'. A more valid criticism of the proposal lies in its possible effects on the foetus in that a proportion – up to 19 per cent – of very low birthweight, yet salvageable, infants may sustain serious defects purely by virtue of their prematurity,[125] and that such abnormalities may well be undetectable at birth. Any legislation along these lines should therefore be guarded. The following is a suggested wording:

A termination of pregnancy involving a foetus which is likely to be capable of attaining a separate existence is to be carried out, save in an emergency to preserve the life of the mother, with the intention of assisting the abortus to live. In applying treatment to this end, the doctor may take into account the actual physical state of the infant and also the foreseeable effect of prematurity on its future development.

Subject to the mother's agreement, a foetus so saved is to be regarded as an abandoned child and may be offered for adoption.

It would, of course, be held that complications of the abortion law such as are proposed here would be difficult to understand and would compromise the physician's clinical independence; and the experience of somewhat complicated legislation in New Zealand might be cited in support.[126] Nevertheless, it represents an attempt at a compromise aimed to draw the two sides together; and the inherent difficulties might, in fact, be salutary – it is not altogether a bad thing that doctors should sometimes have to pause to consider whether their actions are in accord with the public conscience as it is represented by the law.

There remains the problem of the foetal defect grounds for abortion and the extent to which these should depend upon foetal, as opposed to maternal, rights. Ramsey[127] has distinguished between abortion and what he calls 'foetal euthanasia', and there are some very good reasons why this distinction should be made. The right to choose to live or die in an intolerable or painful situation should surely be allowed to the foetus in the same degree as it is to the neonate or to the adult human being. Certainly, any such right can only be exercised in surrogate fashion – through the foetus' parents or medical attendants – but such life and death decisions should be made with the interests of the *foetus* as the primary concern. Clarifying foetal rights in this way would also make 'wrongful life' actions available and would limit the manifest inequity which now bars such suits – the foetus in an action such as *McKay*[128] would be able to claim that it was he or she who was negligently denied a choice to die or to live in misery and the difficult problems of causation would thus be largely eliminated.

On the other hand, the right of the mother to retain her defective infant should never be denied and, again, suitable legislation would not be easy to fashion. One possibility is, first, to ensure the intentions of the Abortion Act 1967, s. 1(1)(b) – the 'foetal grounds' – by adding an explanatory sentence: ' . . . and that, as a result, its quality of life would be severely compromised' and, then, to qualify this by:

Such a termination must still be subject to the mother's consent, and,

in the event of refusal in good faith, no action in tort will be available
to the foetus against its mother.

Finally, the likelihood that foetal euthanasia may involve relatively
late foeticide must be accepted. Provisions such as those in the
Infant Life (Preservation) Act 1929 which are designed to protect
the foetus would therefore have to be lifted where they ceased to
operate in the foetal interests. In this respect, the 1987 Bill is unique
among the many attempts at legislative amendment which have
been made in the British Parliament in the last two decades. It
is uncompromising in its intention that the only 'foetal grounds'
justifying late termination would be that the child was likely to be
born dead or with physical abnormalities so serious that its life
could not be independently sustained, which does no more than
offer the non-viable foetus a choice as to its mode of death.
Although diagnostic techniques are improving rapidly, it remains
true that many foetal abnormalities are, of necessity, only recognized later than 18 weeks of gestation; thus the Bill not only fails
to recognize a foetal right to refuse 'treatment' but it also removes
a considerable proportion of such advantages as are, at present,
exercised by its mother. It is extremely unlikely that the Bill will
reach the statute book without substantial alteration.

It must, of course, be acknowledged that no legislation, including
such a compromise as has been suggested above, which admits
abortion as an option, will satisfy those who regard foeticide at
any stage after conception as being morally unacceptable. No-one
doubts the sincerity of such views, nor that they merit considerable
support; the trouble, as always, is that we live in the real world
and not in never-never land.

Notes

1 Amended by the Criminal Law Act 1967, s. 12(5).
2 S. 60 deals with the offence of concealment of birth which is of interest to
   the pathologist in relation to abortion but which will not be discussed further
   in this chapter.
3 Gordon, G. H., *The Criminal Law of Scotland*, 2nd edn, Edinburgh, W. Green &
   Son, 1978. The subject, including discussion of the Abortion Act 1967, occu-
   pies less than three pages.
4 *H. M. Adv.* v. *Semple* 1937 JC 41.
5 Outside the Indian subcontinent, including, *inter alia*, Malaysia and
   Singapore.
6 This was, of course, before birth by caesarian section became a commonplace.
7 *R.* v. *Bourne*, [1939] 1 KB 687, [1983] 3 All ER 615.
8 *R.* v. *Bourne*, [1939] 1 KB, *per* Macnaughten J., at p. 691.
9 Ibid., at pp. 693–4.

10 R. v. *Newton and Stunge*, [1958] Crim. LR 467 and 600.

11 R. v. *Davidson*, [1969] VR, 667.

12 R. v. *Wald*, (1971) 3 DCR (NSW) 25.

13 Ibid., *per* Menhennit J. at p. 672.

14 Crimes Act 1900, ss. 82–84 (NSW); Crimes Act 1958, ss. 65, 66 (Vict.).

15 Criminal Law Consolidation Act 1935–1980, s. 82a (SA) Criminal Law Consolidation Act and Ordinance 1876–1974, s. 79A (NT).

16 Baird, D., 'Induced abortion: epidemiological aspects', 1 *Journal of Med Ethics*, 122, 1975.

17 Finnis, J. M., 'Three schemes of regulation' in Noonan, J. T. (ed.), *The Morality of Abortion*, Harvard University Press, 1970.

18 The non-British reader may be irritated by the frequent references to geographic location but some pedantry is essential. The United Kingdom consists of Great Britain and Northern Ireland but the Abortion Act 1967 does not apply to Northern Ireland. Within Great Britain, Scotland has its own legal system which differs both in form and substance from that of England and Wales. For example, neither the Offences Against the Person Adt 1861 nor the Infant Life (Preservation) Act 1929 run to Scotland. Many statutes are rendered superfluous by the importance of the common law in the Scottish jurisdiction.

19 *Registrar General's Statistical Review of England and Wales for 1967*, Part III, London, HMSO, 1971.

20 Abortion Act 1967 s. 1 (1)(a).

21 George III, Ch. 58, 1803.

22 Keown, I. J., ' "Miscarriage": a medico-legal analysis', *Criminal Law Review*, 604, 1984.

23 A moral case could, for example, be made out for practices which, on the face of it, are reprehensible – for example, abortion on the grounds of foetal sex. For an interesting lay analysis, see Amiel, B., 'Questions of right and wrong', *The Times*, 8 January 1988.

24 In Scotland, a statement on oath by any person to the effect that he or she has a conscientious objection is sufficient evidence for the purpose (s. 4(3)).

25 The fact that a stillbirth must be of 28 weeks' gestation is immaterial to the present discussion. Births and Deaths Registration Act 1953, s. 4; Registration of Births, Deaths and Marriages (Scotland) Act 1965, s. 56.

26 And, in fact, the World Health Organization does offer such a definition.

27 Williams, G., *Textbook of Criminal Law*, 2nd edn., London, Stevens, 1983, p. 290.

28 C. v. *S.*, *The Times*, 24 February 1987 (QBD); 25 February, CA. For discussion, see Dyer, C., 'Father fails in attempt to stop girlfriend's abortion' **294** *British Medical Journal*, 1987, 631.

29 See Shapiro, S. R., 'Validity under Federal Constitution of abortion laws' 35 L Ed 2d 735 (1973).

30 *Roe* v. *Wade*, 93 S Ct 705 (1973); *Doe* v. *Bolton*, 93 S Ct 739 (1973).

31 *American College of Obstetricians and Gynecologists, Pennsylvania Section and others* v. *Thornburgh and others*, 106 S Ct 2169 (1986). A useful summary for the British reader is to be found in Rouse, F., 'Abortion', *Institute of Medical Ethics Bulletin* Supp no. 5, April 1987.

32 O'Neill, P. T. and Watson, I., 'The father and the unborn child', **38** *Modern Law Review*, 1975, 174.

33 note 30, *supra*.

34 *Harris* v. *McRae*, 100 S Ct 2671 (1980).

35 *H. L.* v. *Matheson* 101 S Ct 1164 (1981)] see also *Bellotti* v. *Baird* 443 US 622 (1979) for consideration of an older girl.

36   At least in England and Wales, although the wording of the 1969 Act does seem to imply that consent to treatment given by someone under the age of 16 could also be valid. In Scotland, the position is that there is no fixed age for consent, and that the decision will be taken on the basis of the child's capacity to understand. See Scottish Law Commission, Consultative Memorandum No. 65, *Legal Capacity of Pupils and Minors*.

37   *Gillick* v. *West Norfolk and Wisbech Area Health Authority* [1983] 3 WLR 859, (QBD); [1985] 2 WLR 413, (CA); 3 WLR 830 (HL). See also *Johnson* v. *Wellesley Hospital* (1970) 17 DLR (3rd) 139 for a similar Canadian approach.

38   Consultative Memorandum, note 36, *supra*.

39   *Re P (a Minor)* (1982) 80 LGR 301; see also the Australian case *K* v. *Minister for Youth and Community Service* [1982] 1 NSWLR 311.

40   *In Re B (a Minor) (Sterilisation)* [1987] 2 All ER 206.

41   Gibb, F., *The Times*, 28 May 1987, p. 1.

42   Gunn, M. J., 'Sex and the mentally handicapped: a lawyer's view' **5** *Medical Law*, 1986, 255.

43   As opposed to the powers of wardship which lapse when the ward reaches the age of 18.

44   *In re B (a minor)*, *supra cit.*, *per* Lord Oliver, at p. 218; for an extensive review of the *parens patriae* doctrine, see *Re Eve* (1986) 31 DLR (4th) 1.

45   '*In re X*', *The Times*, 4 June 1987.

46   Order 15, rule 16.

47   '*In Re T.*; *T* v. *T.*', *The Times*, 11 July 1987.

48   For further discussion, see Chapter 6 *infra*.

49   Ely, J. H., 'The wages of crying wolf: a comment on *Roe* v. *Wade*', **82** *Yale Law Journal*, 1973, 920.

50   Havard, J. D. J., 'Therapeutic abortion' *Criminal Law Review*, 600, 1958. The same restrictions may apply in, say, those Australian states which have no enabling legislation.

51   *McKay* v. *Essex Area Health Authority* [1982] 2 WLR 890. Damages were awarded the mother in a similar case, *Rawnsley* v. *Leeds Area Health Authority*', *The Times*, 17 November 1981.

52   For further discussion, see Chapter 4 *infra*.

53   *McKay* v. *Essex Area Health Authority*, op. cit., at p. 902.

54   See Glover, J., *Causing Death and Saving Lives*, Harmondsworth, Penguin, 1977, ch. 11(5) (reprinted 1986).

55   See Chapter 3 *infra*. For a recent overview see Mason, J. K. and Meyers, D. W., 'Parental choice and selective non-treatment of deformed newborns: a view from mid-Atlantic' **12** *Journal of Medical Ethics*, 67, 1986.

56   *Emeh* v. *Kensington and Chelsea and Westminster Area Health Authority* [1985] 2 WLR 233.

57   Ibid., *per* Slade LJ at pp. 243–4.

58   A precise but variable time is stated in many Commonwealth legislations – for example, 20 weeks (India and New Zealand), 23 weeks (Australia NT), 24 weeks (Singapore).

59   In *Paton* v. *Trustees of the British Pregnancy Advisory Service* [1978] 2 All ER 987. *Borowski* v. *A-G of Canada et al* (1984) 4 DLR (4th) 121 is a recent restatement.

60   Other early moments such as segmentation of the early embryo or the development of recognizable neural tissue have been suggested but are scarcely relevant to abortion.

61   I have argued my reasons for this at length elsewhere and this is an inappropriate point at which to reproduce a discussion which is more theoretical than practical. See, for example, Mason J. K., *Human Life and Medical Practice*, Edinburgh, University Press, 1988, ch. 7.

62 Note 28, *supra*.
63 See the seminal cases of *Watt* v. *Rama* [1972] VR 353; *Duval* v. *Seguin* [1972] 26 DLR (3d) 418; or the early US decision *Bonbrest* v. *Kotz* 65 F Supp 138 (1946); Congenital Disabilities (Civil Liability) Act 1976 (England and Wales); Scottish Law Commission, *Liability for Ante-Natal Injury*, Cmnd. 5371, 1973.
64 For review, see Keyserlingk, E. W., 'A right of the unborn child to prenatal care – the civil law perspective', 13 *Revue de Droit*, 1982, 49; Bartholomew, G., 'The unborn baby and the law' in *Proceedings of the 6th World Congress on Medical Law*, 1982, Ghent, vol 2, p. 53 is most valuable but, unfortunately, an obscure reference. See also the US cases *Bennett* v. *Hymers* 147 A 2d 108 (NH. 1958); *Presley* v. *Newport Hospital* 365 A 2d 748 (RI, 1976).
65 Note 30, *supra*.
66 *Jefferson* v. *Griffin Spalding County Hospital Authority* 274 SE 2d 457 (Ga. 1981).
67 *Raleigh Pitkin-Paul Morgan Memorial Hospital* v. *Anderson* 201 A 2d 537 (NJ, 1964).
68 *Taft* v. *Taft*, 446 NE 2d 395 (Mass. 1983).
69 Ibid., at p. 397.
70 Craft, I., 'When a code catches out the childless', *The Times*, 24 September 1987. There is an excellent account of foetal–patients' rights in Lenow, J. L., 'The fetus as a patient: Emerging rights as a person?' 9 *American Journal of Medical Law*, 1983, 1; see also Callahan, D., 'How technology is reframing the abortion debate', *Hastings Center Report*, 1986, pp. 33–42.
71 Note 59, *supra*, see also in the US *Coe* v. *Gerstein* 41 L Ed 2d 68 (1973).
72 *Paton* v. *United Kingdom* (1980) 3 EHRR 408.
73 *Planned Parenthood of Central Missouri* v. *Danforth* 428 US 52 (1976); *Doe* v. *Doe* 314 NE 2d 128 (Mass. 1974).
74 Note 28, *supra*.
75 A similar distinction was made in *Doe supra cit.*, note 73.
76 Yorke, D. M., 'The legal personality of the unborn child', *Scots Law Times*, 1979, p. 158.
77 *Dehlen* v. *Ottawa Civic Hospital*, (1980) 101 DLR (3d) 686; (1981) 117 DLR (3d) 512.
78 *Re Simms and H* (1979) 106 DLR (3d) 435.
79 *Borowski* v. *Attorney-General of Canada* [1987] 4 WWR 285 (Sask., CA)
80 Note 54, *supra*., ch. 11(3).
81 Note 80, *supra*., at p. 283.
82 *Royal College of Nursing of the United Kingdom* v. *Department of Health and Social Security* [1981] 2 WLR 279, CA and HL.
83 *R* v. *Salford Health Authority, ex parte Janaway'*, *The Times*, 13 February 1987.
84 The decision was affirmed in the Court of Appeal, reported in *The Times*, 5 January 1988. Nevertheless, leave to appeal to the House of Lords was granted.
85 See a predictive analysis by Lafitte, F., 'Recent and possible future trends in abortion', 4 *Journal of Medical Ethics*, 1978, p. 25.
86 *Morgentaler, Smolin and Scott* v. *Her Majesty and A-G of Canada* Supreme Court of Canada, 28 January 1988.
87 *Borowski* note 79, *supra*. Leave to appeal to the Supreme Court granted.
88 For discussion, see Knoppers, B. M., 'Comparative abortion law; the living abortus' in Mason, J. K. (ed.), *Paediatric Forensic Medicine*, London, Chapman Hall, 1988, ch. 25.
89 There were 92,000 deaths at Hiroshima and there are 150,000 abortions annually in the Federal German Republic. See Esser, W., 'Can abortion be legally justified?', 3, *Medical Law*, 1984, p. 205.
90 *R* v. *Smith (John)* [1974] 1 All ER 376.

91   In 1966, the last year before the passing of the Abortion Act, 62 illegal abortionists were brought to jury trial; 22 of them received prison sentences. Four non-professional persons were found guilty under the Offences Against the Person Act 1861, s. 58 in 1983.

92   Lane Committee, *Report of the Committee on the Working of the Abortion Act* (Mrs Justice Lane, chairman) Cmnd. 5579, 1974.

93   There is statistical evidence to show that this has a marked effect. The ratio of resident–non-resident abortions in England and Wales was 2.05:1 in 1974; this rose to 4.59:1 in 1985.

94   *Faridian* v. *General Medical Council* [1970] 3 WLR 1065.

95   *Tarnesby* v. *Kensington, Chelsea and Westminster Area Health Authority* [1980] 1CR 475 (CA); [1981] IRLR 369 (HL).

96   'No case for an abortion Bill' (editorial), **2** *British Medical Journal*, 1979, 230.

97   Brahams, D., 'Putting *Arthur's* case in perspective', *Criminal Law Review*, 1986, 387.

98   Yu, U. Y. H. *et al.*, 'Prognosis for infants born at 23 to 28 weeks' gestation, **293**, *British Medical Journal* 1986, 1200.

99   Lord Wells-Pestell, 355 HL Official Report (5th series), col. 776 (12 December 1974).

100   Williams. op. cit., note 27 *supra.*, p. 292.

101   Tunkel, V., 'Abortion: how early, how late, and how legal?', **2** *British Medical Journal*, 1979, 253.

102   Note 86, *supra.*

103   Ibid., at para 278.

104   Somerville, M. A., 'Reflections on Canadian abortion law: evacuation and destruction – two separate issues', **31** *U Toronto Law Journal*, 1981, 1.

105   *Commonwealth* v. *Edelin*, 359 NE 2d 4 (Mass. 1976).

106   See Towers, B., 'The trials of Dr Waddill', **5** *Journal of Medical Ethics*, 1979, 205.

107   Inquest on Infant Campbell, Stoke-on-Trent, 19 October 1963.

108   '*R* v. *Hamilton*', *The Times*, 16 September 1983.

109   'Bishop throws in the towel', *Guardian*, 12 February 1987, referring to the withdrawal of the Infant Life (Preservation) Bill 1987. For further discussion see Wright, G., 'The legality of abortion by prostaglandin' *Criminal Law Review*, 1984, 347; Tunkel, V., 'Late abortions and the crime of child destruction: (1) A reply', *Criminal Law Review*, 1985, 133.

110   Gordon, *op. cit.*, note 3 *supra.*

111   *H.M. Adv.* v. *Anderson* 1928 JC 1; see also *H.M. Adv.* v. *Semple, supra cit.*, note 4.

112   Keown, I. J., ' "Miscarriage": a medico-legal analysis', *Criminal Law Review*,1984, p. 604.

113   Williams, G., 'Human Life and post-coital pill', *The Times*, 13 April 1983, p. 11.

114   *The Times*, 11 May 1983.

115   Note 86, *supra*, para 91. For discussion, see Tunkel, *op. cit.* note 95, supra.

116   See Chapter 2 *supra.*

117   For discussion, see Keown, J., 'Selective reduction of multiple pregnancy' **137** *New Law Journal*, 1987, 1165.

118   It now is in parts of the USA. See *Justus* v. *Atchison* 565 P 2d. 122 (Cal. 1977)

119   See Craft, I., 'When a code catches out the childless', *The Times*, 24 September 1987.

120   Attitudes have probably not changed greatly since the time of *R.* v. *Dudley & Stephens* (1884) 14 QBD 273.

121   The Second Report of the Voluntary Licensing Authority for Human *in vitro*

Fertilization and Embryology (1987) considers that not more than three pre-embryos should be transferred in any one cycle, unless there are exceptional circumstances – in which case, up to four may be transferred (Guideline 12a)

122 See Callahan, *loc. cit.*, note 65, *supra*.

123 This is, essentially, a restatement of ideas which are promulgated elsewhere in a different context: Mason, op. cit., note 60, *supra.*, chs 7 and 9.

124 *Colautti* v. *Franklin* 439 US 379 (1979); *American College of Obstetricians and Gynecologists et al, supra cit.* note 31.

125 Yu, V. Y. H., 'The extremely low birthweight infant: ethical issues in treatment', **23** *Australian Paediatrics Journal*, 1987, 97.

126 The abortion rate in New Zealand is one of the lowest in the developed countries. The system, involving certifying consultants and regional counsellors (Contraception, Sterilisation and Abortion Act 1977) results in over 80 per cent of terminations being performed in the four main metropolitan cities of New Zealand but there is no reason to suppose that this is a major factor influencing the rate. See *Report of the Abortion Supervisory Committee* for the year ended March 1986.

127 Ramsey, P., 'Reference points in deciding about abortion' in Noonan, J. T. (ed.), *The Morality of Abortion*, Harvard University Press, 1970.

128 *Supra cit.*, note 51.

4 Wrongful birth and life, wrongful death before birth, and wrongful law

BERNARD DICKENS

Introduction

It is trite to observe that the law of torts or delict, which aim primarily to oblige wrongdoers to make monetary or other compensation to those they injure, and thereby to deter injury, do not evolve in a vacuum. Historians explain the influences that have given tort law its modern contours, but what should influence its future is argued by trial lawyers, politicians, academic commentators on law, ethics, economy and a range of related disciplines, and lay people. Activist groups, of whatever composition and orientation, contend that the law should take or retain a particular form because that would accord to their general vision of justice, or because that form would serve a specific goal or interest favoured by the group. An instrumental approach to tort law, taken in order that the law may further a preferred result and deny or obstruct a disfavoured result, is not uncommon even among groups that invoke absolutist rather than consequentialist or utilitarian values.

The field of medical law has been strongly animated in the last few decades by the debate over abortion. Although this originated as a debate on the proper social role and function of criminal law, the criminal abortion issue quickly expanded into adjacent areas of the law, and came to affect the field of tort law as well as family law.[1] With improvements in medical care, in reliability of contraceptive means and in access to voluntary sterilization to limit life-endangering pregnancies, and with women's increasing recourse to qualified practitioners to perform abortion following decriminalization, maternal mortality[2] has declined in developed countries. Accordingly, the issue of sanctity of human life in the abortion debate has come to focus less on prospective danger to pregnant women's lives than on the clear danger abortion presents to foetuses.[3]

Medical advances have also developed knowledge of genetic and other congenital sources of danger to children's health, which has produced predictive tests of both prospective parents and foetuses. Further, means have been created not only to offer genetic and other counselling of prospective parents, both before and after conception, but also to relieve certain of the conditions that prejudice the birth of healthy children. More recently, surgical means have been developed to treat certain foetal ailments *in utero*, and even to remove a foetus from the womb for treatment and then to return it to continue gestation there.[4] Now that the foetus is visible, tangible and treatable, whether *in utero* or *extra uterum*, it has acquired the status of a patient in medicine, although in traditional common law it may lack status as a human being.[5]

Opposing ends of the philosophical spectrum on the abortion issue are occupied by those who describe themselves as being 'Pro-Life' and 'Pro-Choice'. The former oppose the legalization of abortion under all circumstances, or all but those in which pregnant women face clear danger to their lives or perhaps serious danger to their permanent health. The latter oppose any criminalization of abortion and favour women's freedom to decide whether to continue or terminate pregnancy without legal prescription. The legally derived concept of a 'human being' and the legal and ethical concepts of 'a person' and 'personhood' have been drawn into the abortion debate regarding the status to be given to, or inherent in, the foetus.[6]

A colonizing effect of the abortion controversy, particularly in the USA, has been Pro-Life hostility to success of tort actions by parents of handicapped children claiming that they were wrongfully denied medical recourse to abortion, and to actions by children themselves claiming that they should have been aborted. These claims are seen to do violence to the sanctity of human life and to give medical professionals incentives to recommend and to perform abortions lest they may bear legal liability following birth. Lobbying in a few US jurisdictions has resulted in legislation that removes tortious liability for any negligent act or omission that results in a child's birth. Against this, the Pro-Life movement urges tortious liability for negligent conduct causing foetal loss, and legal recognition of foetal personhood through which action may be taken on behalf of the stillborn foetus itself.

The Pro-Choice position is sympathetic to actions by parents for wrongful denial of the option of abortion, and to actions by those choosing to have children who suffer foetal loss due to another's fault. Foetal personhood tends to be opposed not so much in itself, but for the limiting effect it may have, and is indeed often intended to have, on the availability of abortion services.

This study argues that the Pro-Life position should be legally rejected in the development of tort law, because it seeks to deny compensation to children born alive with handicaps but to provide compensation to foetuses that are not born alive. It is argued instead that children suffering pain and medical costs due to others' wrongful conduct should be entitled to compensation, and that negligence that results in foetal loss can be properly compensated and deterred by legal means other than by compelling payments to be made to the estates of stillborn foetuses. Those who suffer lost opportunities to have the children they want should be entitled to a cause of action against anyone whose negligence or other wrong is alleged to have caused the loss. Further, it argues that tort law development should not be confused, distorted or manipulated to score symbolic points or make advances in the abortion conflict, or to serve the agenda of any protagonist in this controversy that is only marginally related to the law of compensation.

Reproduction law has generated a variety of related legal claims described by labels that tend to be confused or, from the perspective of advocates of particular nomenclatures, misapplied. Misdescriptions have been applied by successful advocates of claims and appear in influential judgements, so that the actual nature of a claim or principle of decision can be difficult to ascertain unless the specific facts of an individual case are studied. However, intensive scholarly US literature shows that, in recent times, a settled and widely agreed system of differentiation has come to be accepted.[7] This system, which is adopted hereafter, provides that:

- *Wrongful pregnancy* is a claim that another's negligence resulted in a plaintiff's unplanned conception of a child, whether or not the pregnancy was carried to term.
- *Wrongful conception* is a narrower claim that negligent performance of a sterilization procedure resulted in a conception which the purportedly sterilized plaintiff intended should not occur, but no child was born due to spontaneous or induced abortion;
- *Wrongful birth* is a claim that a health care provider violated a legal duty owed to a parent to give information or to perform a medical procedure with due care, resulting in the birth of a defective child:
- *Wrongful life* is a claim by, or on behalf of, a person born with predictable physical or mental handicaps that, but for the defendant's negligence, the person would not have been

conceived or, having been conceived, would not have been born alive;

● *Dissatisfied life* is a claim by, or on behalf of, a person that he or she was born with disadvantages of a non-medical nature due to a defendant's wrong, such as the disadvantage of being illegitimate.[8]

A wrongful life action is different from a routine claim for prenatal injury that seeks damages because, in the latter, but for the defendant's negligence, an injured person would have existed without the injury the defendant is alleged to have caused. The essence of the wrongful life claim is that, but for the defendant's wrong, the person would never have been conceived or born.

Wrongful birth

The wrongful birth action is invoked only when a defective child is born. In the case of the birth of a healthy but unplanned child, the cause of action is for wrongful pregnancy. The wrongful pregnancy action itself has historically attracted judicial and wider opposition, perhaps on intuitive or aesthetic grounds, since it implies that the birth of a healthy though unplanned child is a species of legal injury. With the decline of the view that a child's birth is a divine gift, and the prevalence of the view that it is an event that parents can, and should, plan responsibly, many courts have rejected the approach that a child's birth is an unmixed blessing. They have accepted that a reasonable balance can be struck between the benefits and the burdens of childbirth, and that, when the latter are excessive in a particular case, compensation may properly be awarded when negligence has been shown. A long-standing cultural assumption that the birth of a healthy child is always a blessing continues to be invoked in doctrinaire jurisprudence,[9] but a preferably pragmatic observation was made in the Michigan Court of Appeal in 1971 that:

> Contraceptives are used to prevent the birth of healthy children. To say that for reasons of public policy contraceptive failure can result in no damage as a matter of law ignores the fact that tens of millions of persons use contraceptives daily to avoid the very result which the defendant would have us say is always a benefit, never a detriment. Those tens of millions of persons, by their conduct, express the sense of the community.[10]

Nevertheless, damages tend to be denied for costs associated with rearing the child, and are limited to such matters as physical and mental pain and suffering incurred during pregnancy and childbirth, medical expenses incurred during pregnancy and delivery, lost wages and, in the case of negligent sterilization, either a refund of the original costs or the costs associated with a second operation.[11]

The wrongful birth action has now been allowed by the English Court of Appeal[12] consistently with a sizeable volume of common law jurisprudence that has come to recognize the propriety of awarding damages for a parent's extra burden of rearing a handicapped child. The crux of the action is a negligent deprivation of choice. The plaintiffs do not claim that the defendants caused their children to be abnormal or injured. Claims that the defendants caused the plaintiffs' children to be injured when they would otherwise have been born uninjured would be routine tort claims for prenatal harm resulting in avoidable injuries. Rather, wrongful birth claims allege that health care providers' negligence deprived the plaintiffs of information – for example of their genetic prognosis, of the availability of prenatal diagnosis, or of the correct results of prenatal diagnosis necessary for them to make proper choices of whether to conceive children or to continue pregnancies. They claim that, had such information been given, they would not have had the children.

The wrongful birth action developed after biological means of genetic diagnosis and prognosis made it possible to counsel prospective parents on their unconceived children's likely genetic inheritance, and abortion law reform had coincided with developments in prenatal diagnosis, so that those who could be informed of the genetic or other congenital risks facing their conceived children could lawfully act on that information to terminate pregnancies. Success of the claim depended on plaintiffs establishing the four standard elements of a tort claim, namely that a legal duty of care was owed to them, that it was violated by conduct falling short of the legally determined standard of care, that they suffered a species of legally recognized injury, and that the injury was proximately caused by the breach of duty of care.

Developments, particularly in the field of medical genetics, in time persuaded courts to find that duties of warning of genetic and related congenital risks could arise in the healthy professional--patient relationship, and that performance standards could be judicially determined, failure to observe which would constitute breach of that duty. The birth of a defective child was more easily seen to be a legally recognized damage than the birth of a healthy child. The damage was not the child itself but loss of the choice whether to assume the financial and emotional costs of caring for that child, that exceeded the costs of rearing a normal child. Causation was demonstrable on evidence either that the appropriately informed plaintiff would probably not have conceived the child – for instance through remaining unmarried or by having resort to sterilization,[13] or that a pregnancy would have been both terminable and terminated. Although litigation is specific to the parties, and particularly to the plaintiff, claims of subjective disposition to avoid a conception are so clearly self-serving that courts tend to seek objective evidence of what a reasonable person is likely to have done in the plaintiff's circumstances, and often speculate about what it is reasonable to expect and require people in general to do.

The first case to give prominence to the wrongful birth claim in the common law world involved a woman in New Jersey, who contracted rubella (German measles) early in pregnancy. She claimed that she informed her doctor of this fact, but that he gave her no warning of the danger the disease posed to the development of the foetus. Abortion was generally illegal in New Jersey at that time, although it was lawfully available to the plaintiff parent nearby in New York State. The court in 1967 rejected the claim partly on the abortion issue,[14] invoking the public policy consideration that the state's prohibition of abortion precluded an award of damages for loss of the opportunity to undergo the procedure.

In addition, however, the New Jersey court invoked the impossibility of measuring damages for which the plaintiff parents sought compensation. It was reasoned that:

> In order to determine their compensatory damages a court would have to evaluate the denial to them of the intangible, unmeasurable, and complex human benefits of motherhood and fatherhood and weigh these against the alleged emotional and money injuries. . . . When the parents say their child should not have been born, they make it impossible for a court to measure their damages in being the mother and father of a defective child.[15]

A dissenting judgement in the case observed that the prevailing majority judgment ' . . . permits a wrong with serious consequential injury to go wholly unredressed',[16] and contended that courts which daily evaluate such intangible, unmeasurable and complex human experiences as pain, suffering, humiliation and betrayal are able to evaluate the harm caused by wrongful birth.

This dissenting approach to the claim was favoured by many commentators in the years following 1967, and was reinforced by the 1973 US Supreme Court ruling that such state prohibition of access to abortion was unconstitutional in most cases.[17] Indeed, it has been documented in the US that:

Following the *Gleitman* decision, no other court accepted the *Gleitman* rationale regarding wrongful birth. By contrast, every court that has considered the issue since *Gleitman* has chosen to recognize the wrongful birth action.[18]

Courts in other common law jurisdictions have similarly found that routine tort principles allow the action, and that no principles of public policy prevent its recognition. The Victoria, Australia, case of *Watt* v. *Rama*[19] was an early instance, but modern examples exist in England[20] and, for instance, Canada.[21] In *Zimmer* v. *Ringrose*[22] in Alberta, Canada, moreover, damages were awarded against a doctor whose follow-up care after sterilization was inadequate in assisting his pregnant patient to seek an abortion.[23]

This raises the sensitive issue of whether a woman who has a wrongful pregnancy is obliged to mitigate her injury, as plaintiffs generally are, to the extent of precluding a wrongful birth claim by having an abortion if it is medically favourable for her, or by giving up the child for adoption if abortion is contra-indicated – for instance due to advanced gestation. It seems unlikely that judges, recognizing a woman's legal right to have an abortion, would go so far as to impose a duty to abort, owed to a liable defendant, by way of mitigation of damages. In the 'Emeh' case,[24] however, the trial judge confined damages in a wrongful birth claim to those relevant to a wrongful pregnancy claim – that is for sickness and the distress of four months of pregnancy – because he considered that, at that point, the plaintiff's rejection of the available abortion option evidenced her new intention to keep the child. The judge said of Mrs Emeh that:

> . . . . her own unacceptable reasons for not seeking an abortion have convinced me that, in truth, she elected to allow the pregnancy to continue because she wanted to bear another child, and from that time onwards her pregnancy was not unwanted.[25]

The Court of Appeal did not accept this interpretation of Mrs Emeh's motivation, however, and found that it was reasonable for her to decline abortion at the stage of pregnancy she had reached on grounds of her own health.[26] On the matter of principle, moreover, Slade L. J. observed that, save in the most exceptional of circumstances, 'I cannot think it right that the court should ever declare it unreasonable for a woman to decline to have an abortion'.[27]

This principle is in accordance with commonly prevailing jurisprudence, which considers that no woman should be expected to mitigate damages by recourse to abortion or adoption, or be disadvantaged in compensation for refusal to use these options where they exist. In 1971 the Michigan Court of Appeal summarized the principle that:

> The defendant does not have the right to insist that the victim of his negligence have the emotional and mental makeup of a woman who is willing to abort or place a child for adoption.[28]

The Pro-Life movement clearly favours the principle, and the Pro-Choice movement supports women's autonomous choice both not to have and also to have children.

In the same way that many jurisdictions decline to award damages in wrongful pregnancy cases for the costs of raising a healthy child,[29] many courts in wrongful birth cases decline to award full recovery for costs of rearing a handicapped child. They limit damages to calculated expenses that exceed those normally involved in childrearing. When the child's defects and disabilities are severe, these can be very considerable indeed – unless, of course, the child's lifespan is expected to be limited.[30] This basis of compensation is appropriate, perhaps, where parents intend to have a normal child, but not the handicapped child they conceive due to a defendant's negligence. When they are wrongfully denied a legal opportunity to abort, however, they may reasonably expect full compensation, because they have been denied their entitlement to have no child. The same is even more true when plaintiffs intend not to be parents at all, but become parents of a handicapped child due to negligent contraceptive care or the negligent conduct, for instance, of a sterilization or abortion procedure.

Underlying judicial refusal to award damages to cover costs of rearing a healthy child, whether in wrongful pregnancy cases or in wrongful birth cases where only excess costs are allowed in damages, is the view that all human life is a gift or blessing – a view which is sometimes articulated in judgements. However, this celebration of children denies the compatible social and legal reality that many conscientious, responsible couples do not want children, either at all or at particular times. The achievement through modernization of criminal law and otherwise of legislated, judicially declared and constitutionally protected rights of lawful resort to contraception, voluntary sterilization and abortion shows this, even to those to whom these options are personally and publicly objectionable.

The common law system often permits judges excessive licence to indulge their personal intuitions and idiosyncratic fantasies, and to present their individual perceptions and sentiments as social truths and principles of public policy. Whether or not births of children into families in particular circumstances amount to blessings does not have to be determined by judges' untutored instincts. The issue is amenable to the presentation of evidence from social scientists and of, for instance, demographic health and family-functioning data. Such evidence may not be comprehensive or unambiguous, of course, but the conclusions to be drawn from it would be exposed to adversarial scrutiny, and would suitably displace the unexplained speculation of lawyers and judges.

An example of such *a priori* speculation arose in the 1978 Ontario (Canada) case of *Doiron* v. *Orr*[31] The judge found that a sterilization procedure had not been negligently conducted and dismissed the wrongful pregnancy claim. In case an appeal court should reverse this finding, however, he went on to determine what damages should be awarded, including on the claim of damages for support of the healthy child. Speaking *obiter*, Mr Justice Garrett said:

> . . . personally, I find this approach to a matter of this kind which deals with human life, the happiness of the child, the effect upon its thinking, upon its mind when it realizes that there has been a case of this kind, that it is an unwanted mistake, and that its rearing is being paid for by someone other than its parents, is just simply grotesque.[32]

No relevant case law had been cited to the judge on the issue and his resort to personal sentiment to determine the issue was explicit. In the adjacent Canadian province of Quebec at the same time as the Ontario judgement was being given, a judge of equal status found that a sterilization had been performed negligently and applied routine principles to assess damages that included an albeit modest amount for child support.[33] Similarly, in *Thake* v. *Maurice*, Mr Justice Pain said:

> I do not think that if I award damages here it will lead little Samantha to feel rejection . . . by the time she comes to consider this judgment (if she ever does) she will, I think, welcome it as a means of having made life somewhat easier for her family.[34]

Whether a child will in fact suffer rejection as a result of learning that it was the unwanted result of, for instance, negligent steriliz-ation of a parent, may be doubted if it knows that its parents refused the option of abortion or adoption. Since it is the parents' insistence on raising the child within their family that gives rise to the action, the child has evidence that it is wanted. In any event, however, the issue need not be left to speculation. Studies have been conducted and research can be sponsored – for instance by law reform agencies and family court clinics – on the effects on children of learning that they were conceived through contraception or sterilization failure or, for instance, that they were born as a result of denied abortion. Studies might be directed not just to admission or quantification of damage claims, but also to offering counselling on how best to inform children of such origins. Similarly, enough children are reared at the expense of someone they consider a stranger, such as by maintenance payments made by another's divorced husband, for empirical data to be available on the effect this knowledge has on them.

In *Thake* v. *Maurice*, Mr Justice Pain observed:

> I do not accept that it is a part of our culture that the birth of a child is always a blessing. It may have been the assumption in the past. I feel quite satisfied that it is not the assumption today.[35]

Even if it is accepted, however, that birth of a child is a blessing, it does not follow that it should not be the subject of damages representing costs of childrearing. One commentator has correctly noted that:

> No court would be moved by the argument coming from a putative father that he should not be required to provide financial support for the child he has fathered on the grounds that he has bestowed on the mother a priceless blessing.[36]

It may be observed, of course, that the right of maintenance is the child's and not the mother's, but the child may still regard the payment as symbolizing that he or she is an unwanted mistake, and that its rearing is being paid for by someone it does not consider a social or psychological parent.[37] Mr Justice Garrett found this 'just simply grotesque',[38] but paternity payments in this circumstance have become basic to modern legal systems, and are faulted, not for existing, but for being inadequately enforced.

Further, as a matter of legal doctrine, individuals are entitled to resist the imposition or award of benefits. The sentimental view that childbirth is a benefit that outweighs all economic or other detriments pays insufficient regard to the autonomous legal capacity to decline benefits. Long before evolution of the modern perception that whether or not an experience is a benefit should be assessed by the adult competent subject of that experience, rather than by the perpetrator or a court of law, it was an acknowledged equitable principle that:

> No one has a right to compel another to have his property improved in a particular manner; it is as illegal to force him to receive a benefit as to submit to an injury.[39]

For a court to insist that what a plaintiff considers an injury is in fact a benefit is patronizing and insulting. Even if a court finds no injury in law in a child's birth, it would maintain the plaintiff's dignity and its own credibility by not describing as a benefit what so many make efforts to avoid.

A view similarly dismissive of medical patients' personal and legal powers of autonomy underlies a peculiarly influential argument against allowing wrongful birth actions. In such cases as *McKay* v. *Essex Area Health Authority*[40] and *Udale*[41] reliance was placed by both defendants and the courts on the argument that, if the birth of a child following medical negligence were compensable, doctors would have incentives or pressures to urge and perform abortions. The English Law Commission's *Report on Injuries to Unborn Children* was cited, which states that:

> Such a cause of action, if it existed, would place an almost intolerable burden on medical advisers in their socially and morally exacting role. The danger that doctors would be under subconscious pressures to advise abortions in doubtful cases through fear of an action for damages is, we think, a real one.[42]

The Law Commission was addressing the cause of action for wrongful life, not for wrongful birth, and its application in the Udale case seems misconceived. Indeed, the very next sentence following that quoted above is: 'It must not be forgotten that in certain circumstances, the parents themselves might have a claim in negligence.'[43] The Law Commission apparently did not consider that the argument that doctors facing damage awards on the birth of a child would advise abortion should preclude wrongful birth or, indeed, wrongful pregnancy actions.

The argument has force only if it is accepted that doctors' advice and preferences govern patients' decisions. This view may have weight in the UK, where a relatively high level of medical paternalism remains prevalent and the House of Lords has upheld standards of doctors' disclosure to patients that may deny them information necessary for their due exercise of autonomy.[44] In North America, however, the Supreme Court of Canada has subscribed to modern decisions from the USA on informed consent.[45] These are designed to place patients in control of the commanding heights of medical decisions that affect them, and give them control of the goals of treatment even when they yield choice of means of treatment to doctors. Particularly in the USA, a woman's decision whether to have an abortion is insulated from any decisive or overreaching medical influence.

The argument that wrongful birth damages lead to medically

advised abortion and should therefore be precluded by judicial declaration or legislation has been adopted by the Pro-Life movement. In the USA, successful lobbying to this effect has resulted in state legislatures in Minnesota, Missouri and Utah passing laws which disallow wrongful birth suits.[46] Minnesota's law was subsequently declared to be constitutional and not a denial of the due process right to legal redress,[47] and those of Missouri and Utah are as yet untested. The major objection to the laws and the argument on which they are based remains, however, that they disregard personal autonomy in abortion.

Where those presented with an unwanted pregnancy and/or the risk of having to rear a handicapped child know that they have no legal entitlement to compensation from negligent health care providers, they may use their legal or *de facto* powers to have an abortion. That is, more likely to lead to abortions than the defendants' liability to pay damages for negligence resulting in childbirth, is the plaintiffs' liability to recover damages. The view already exists – which is fearful to some, particularly those in the Pro-Life movement – that parents of handicapped children may order that they not be treated so that death results. In the USA the so-called 'Baby Doe' regulations, subsequently held invalid by the US Supreme Court[48] were promulgated partly in the belief that parents want to avoid the burdens of supporting handicapped children in financial and other ways. Even if the argument that court awards of damages against health professionals cause abortions can be anecdotally or statistically shown to be valid, it is at best quantitatively ambivalent in view of the alternative argument that denial of damages causes parents to abort, and an unsound basis in itself for legislative or judicial policy.

Wrongful life

The wrongful life action, brought by or on behalf of a handicapped child, was named as a derisive and dismissive parody of the wrongful death action, and is currently accepted in only a handful of US jurisdictions. About twenty states' courts have rejected the action.[49] It is interesting to observe, however, that New Jersey, which gave prominence in the 1967 case of *Gleitman* v. *Cosgrove*[50] not only to the wrongful birth claim but also to the wrongful life claim, and comprehensively rejected it, accepted the cause of action in 1984 and overruled Gleitman.[51] Nevertheless, the number of states which have legislatively prohibited the action may soon exceed the number of those judicially accepting it.[52]

The New Jersey Supreme Court in the Gleitman case, where the child plaintiff was born deaf, mute and almost blind, found his claim that he should not have been born but should have been aborted, almost incomprehensible. The Court said:

> The infant plaintiff would have us measure the difference between his life with defects against the utter void of non-existence, but it is impossible to make such a determination. This Court cannot weigh the value of life with impairments against the nonexistence of life itself. By asserting that he should not have been born, the infant plaintiff makes it logically impossible for a court to measure his alleged damages because of the impossibility of making the comparison required by compensatory remedies.[53]

This frequently invoked finding of impossible calculation is subject to the same criticism as that which was made of the Court's finding that a wrongful birth claim was impossible to calculate.[54] The few jurisdictions to have recognized the claim have found means to assess compensation, and academic literature has provided a number of bases of calculation.[55] In rejecting a handicapped child's action, the English Law Commission nevertheless observed:

> Nor would it be easy to assess his damages on any logical basis for it would be difficult to establish a norm with which the plaintiff in his disabled state could be compared. . . . Law is an artefact and, if social justice requires that there should be a remedy given for a wrong, then logic should not stand in the way. A measure of damages could be artificially constructed.[56]

A claim of social justice can be established,[57] although US jurisdictions have rejected the action on a variety of grounds, most of which have stepped beyond traditional legal doctrine and have invoked visions of public policy. The cases raise the separate issue of the proper interaction of judicial and political development of the law. They affect the proactive–reactive conflict of whether courts should decline initiatives to recognize new claims and leave their accommodation to politically composed legislatures, or advance the law where they consider justice requires it and leave legislatures to react on behalf of the societies they represent.

Defence advocates and courts often employ elegant rhetoric and invoke noble sentiments to explain why pitifully handicapped children born due to the professional negligence of health care practitioners have not suffered legal injury. They assert that allowing a wrongful life claim implies that non-existence can be preferable to human life in an impaired condition, and repudiate this idea as an objectionable disavowal of the sanctity of human life and of the unique worth of all human beings. Many variants are made of the theme of human life as an overwhelming and transcending blessing contrasted with which individual pain, suffering, gross handicap or insentience are inconsequential. However, the 'blessing balloon' that was busted several years ago in wrongful pregnancy and wrongful birth claims[58] is now being busted again in wrongful life claims. Courts are increasingly '. . . unwilling to say as a matter of law that life, even with the most severe and debilitating of impairments, is always preferable to non-existence'.[59]

New Jersey courts were aided in the transition from *Gleitman* to *Procanik* v. *Cillo*[60] by being the forum of the case of Karen Quinlan.[61] This celebrated case on the so-called 'right to die' forced recognition, and induced sensitivity, that there are conditions of human life to which death – that is, non-existence – may be preferable. Courts have invoked the sanctity of human life rather than its blessing to resist claims of the right to die. Increasingly, however, particularly when patients suffer major disabilities and loss of cognitive function, US courts recognize that prevention of pain and suffering through allowance of expiration of life is a legitimate goal of medical management, and that cessation of life can be in patients' own best interests. Indeed, it is interesting to speculate whether the real future of the wrongful life action may lie in compensating handicapped children, but in compensating adults denied non-existence through death when life-sustaining treatment is administered over their objections.

Some courts, which have neither eulogized human life nor wilted before the challenge of assessing damages, have nevertheless rejected wrongful life claims on the grounds of basic tort law doctrine. They have concluded that any negligence could violate no duty of care owed to the child-plaintiff, as opposed to its parents. The plaintiff may have been not only unborn at the time, but not yet conceived. There is evident difficulty in a plaintiff's argument that a duty of care was owed to a non-existent person to ensure that he or she should never exist, and that birth proves breach of that duty. Courts sustaining the action have held, however, that a duty may extend to persons unborn or unconceived at the time of the negligent act or omission. This duty is limited by the foreseeability test. It is a regular propositon of tort law that there can be special relationships in which a duty of care is owed to a third person one foresees or reasonably should foresee being injured through one's act or omission.[62] Since the duty is owed to those in a general category and not to a specific individual, one to whom the duty is owed need therefore not be born or conceived at the time of its breach. The consequent damage to a person can accrue some time after the breach, provided that it is proximately caused by the breach. The relation between a health care professional and a patient can create a special relationship and legal duty to children whom it is foreseen the patient may later conceive.[63]

In a wrongful life case, the duty may consist of appropriately informing a patient through genetic or prenatal diagnosis that a child may be conceived or born with severe handicaps, but it is not dependent on sophisticated biotechnology. The obligation may consist of a general duty to observe the standard of care in routine prenatal treatment. Some courts have declined to accept wrongful life because they associate it with sophisticated medical techniques they consider to be beyond judicial administrability.[64] Whilst advanced medical and genetic predictive technologies have certainly given impetus to the action, however, its elements arise from routine medical care.

The causation issue in wrongful life is perhaps one of the least problematic. It is not claimed, of course, that health care professionals caused the plaintiff's congenital injuries. In tort law, a defendant is held to have caused what he or she failed to discharge the duty to prevent. The 'but for' test is routinely applied, which in this case is satisfied if, but for the professional's negligence, the plaintiff's parents would have avoided conception or aborted the pregnancy. In *Harbeson* v. *Parke Davis*,[65] for instance, it was expressly held that a doctor's negligence could be the proximate cause of an infant-plaintiff's injuries where the infant would not have been born had the parents known of the severe foetal abnormalities. The court also observed that allowing the parents' wrongful birth action while denying the infant recovery would be anomalous.

This explains why recognition of wrongful life actions conforms to principles of social justice. Damages in wrongful birth actions may be limited to the extra costs of coping with the child's handicaps, and be limited to the time for which parents are legally bound to care for their children, which may be until they reach 16, 18 or, for instance, 21 years of age. If, exceptionally, a court accepts a parental duty to care for a child not just during minority but during chronic disability, parents may receive damages for the estimated lifespan of the child, either on a lump-sum or annuity basis. Typically, however, parents recover damages to cover only their own responsibilities which expire in time. Thereafter, the adult child must make independent arrangements for support. Further, if parents die before their dependent children's majority, the children's support may end. The issue must be addressed, therefore, of the handicapped child's means of financial support when it reaches adult age or is self-dependent. The wrongful life claim addresses this issue.

Care must be taken that both parent and child do not recover

damages to meet the same support responsibility, but this is relatively easily arranged. In the Harbeson case, the court noted that
the parents' recovery on their wrongful birth action did not include
care for their severely handicapped children after they reached the
age of majority. The children's needs for special medical care, for
nursing attention and for training would continue, however, for all
of their lives. The court considered it just that the burden of these
costs should be placed on those whose negligence caused them.

Rhetoric about the sanctity of life and the symbolic or public
policy goal the law must serve in the celebration of life ignores the
crucial reality that provision must be made for the handicapped.
Pro-Life arguments against the justice of the wrongful life claim
ring particularly hollow in the USA, where niggardly public health
services may leave the handicapped in inadequate or poor care.
Litigation and judicially ordered compensation offer the disadvantaged a humane level of provision that the political system often
denies. In Canada, provincial health insurance plans make available
medical and related services for the handicapped, but they operate
on the usual insurance principles of subrogation, and are interested
to recover their expenditures through injured plaintiffs' litigation
that will make defendants contribute. In the UK, however, there
may be somewhat reduced need for the wrongful life action to be
available to reinforce principles of social justice. If standards of
public provision of health services fall, however, the action may be
necessary for maintenance of individual welfare.

In the McKay case,[66] the three Court of Appeal judges employed
reasoning already familiar in the USA to conclude that the child's
wrongful life action should not be recognized. The facts of the case
arose before the Congenital Disabilities (Civil Liability) Act 1976
came into effect late in July of that year, and the claim was rejected
under the pre-existing common law. The 1976 Act follows
recommendations of the Law Commission made in the Report[67]
which rejected the wrongful life action, principally because of the
suspected tendency to motivate doctors to advise abortions which
would remove their own liability to such suits. In the McKay case
Lord Justice Griffiths took issue with this ground for rejecting the
action, observing that a doctor need fear no liability provided that
he or she adequately explains the risks involved in continuing a
pregnancy – namely that the foetus is abnormal and, if born, would
be a handicapped child. Responsibility for continuation of pregnancy then rests on the parents, whose right to take the risks of
conception and childbirth supersedes any claim their child might
bring against them.[68] The chain of causation linking the doctor to
the handicapped child is broken by this new intervening act of the
informed parents.

The inference from the McKay case and the Law Commission Report that conditioned the Congenital Disabilities (Civil Liability) Act 1976 is that wrongful life actions do not exist under the Act. Respected commentators have noted, however, that a strong argument can be made that the Act does not exclude wrongful life actions, but only governs actions for prenatal injuries.[69] Whatever the position will prove to be, the properly taken objection raised in the McKay case by Lord Justice Griffiths to the primary reason the Law Commission offered for rejecting the action shows how unsatisfactory it is to recommend and enact policies premised on the impact they are believed likely to have on recourse to abortion.[70]

Wrongful death before birth

It seems perverse that in the USA where so many jurisdictions deny wrongful life actions to children born with handicaps due to negligence, many more, including some in the former category, permit recovery on behalf of foetuses which are stillborn due to negligence. The explanation that the former position is a result of judicial declaration of perceived common law principles whilst the latter results from judicial interpretation of legislative language resolves the incongruity only to the satisfaction of the more pedantic of lawyers. To Pro-Life adherents, however, the position is not unsatisfactory, incongruent nor perverse. Wrongful life claims are perceived to cause doctors to favour abortions, and must therefore be opposed, whereas damages awardable to stillborn foetuses encourage the protection of foetal life up to birth. International liaison and shared literature in the Pro-Life movement make it likely that accommodation of claims for wrongful death of foetuses will be urged in jurisdictions where they are not yet common.

Although the issue is initially one of judicial determination of legislative intent, the judicial task can be approached through such a variety of styles – from the extremely conservative to the extremely activist or interventionist – that it warrants attention being given to the principles and implications of their exercise. Indeed, a number of US jurisdictions have observed that such a body of practice has come to rest on the foundation of wrongful death statutes that its development follows the traditions of common law evolution.[71]

Classical common law considered that death was not a civil injury for which compensation could be awarded.[72] Because this made it advantageous for wrongdoers to kill rather than merely injure their victims, legislation was enacted, first in England, providing that wrongdoers were to be as liable to suit on behalf of the deceased whose death they caused as they would have been had death not resulted from their wrong. Lord Campbell's Act – The Fatal Accidents Act 1846 – [73] provided in part that:

> Whensoever the Death of a Person shall be caused by wrongful Act, Neglect, or Default . . . such as would (if Death had not ensued) have entitled the Party injured to maintain an Action and recover Damages . . . The Person who would have been liable if Death had not ensued shall be liable to an Action for Damages, notwithstanding the Death of the Person injured.

Similar language has been employed in many US states, with minor variants in some cases, but with common emphasis on compensating the death of a 'person'. The Pro-Life assertion of the personhood of the unborn has led to the demand that such an Act's reference to a 'person' include the unborn.

A number of advocates and courts favouring this approach take their position, not with regard to its significance in the abortion conflict, but because they find that it does justice to parents who have been denied childbirth through another's negligence. This is a worthy goal to pursue and, in the absence of another cause of action available to such parents, the wrongful death statute is appropriate to use. In fact, however, US jurisdictions have read their wrongful death laws in a wide variety of ways, and even when reading the same type of legislation the same way, often give different and even conflicting reasons for their conclusions. At times, judges on the same bench give quite different explanations of the purpose, scope and effect of their state's legislation. This reflects the immense confusion about what these laws are designed to achieve.

A distinction exists between wrongful death statutes, most of which are modelled on Lord Campbell's Act of 1846 and create a new legal cause of action in the deceased's representative, and survival statutes. The latter overcome the common law principle that any cause of action dies with the person, which disallows posthumously presented or continued claims. The statutes provide instead that whatever cause of action the individual had at death can be litigated on behalf of his or her estate. The distinction may be hard to draw where legislation allows litigation against a wrongdoer whose negligence causes death. A simple survival statute tends not to refer to the cause of death being an accident or wrongful, since it is irrational to provide that a cause of action survives the individual's death only if death was accidental or unnatural. Further, surviving actions are not limited to those for wrongs causing the death. A wrongful death Act on the other hand would afford certain designated persons rights to sue on another's death, in order that their own loss from that death be compensated and that the wrong-doer does not benefit from killing, as opposed to merely injuring, the victim. Modelled on the English 1846 Act, however, much of the legislation prevailing in the USA is unclear, and judicial interpretation tends to increase the margin of uncertainty except insofar as the law becomes settled by precedent within a particular jurisdiction. Indeed, some commentators appear to have become so frustrated in attempts to separate wrongful death from survival statutes regarding the negligent causing of stillbirth that they have contended that the distinction should be ignored and that either type of law be interpreted to include the other.[74]

Much confusion is due to inadequate analysis which focuses on the rights of a 'foetus' itself. A tendency exists to write and speak about legal recognition of the legal rights of a foetus, even while also recognizing that a key condition of the foetus pursuing a right is that it is born alive.[75] Once a foetus is born alive, however, it is in law a human (in) being.[76] and its rights are not dependent on arguments about personhood. Historically, the courts denied claims for prenatal injury,[77] and it was not until 1946 that US courts recognized a person's cause of action for injuries caused *in utero*.[78] The recognized rights are those of born persons, however, and not of foetuses *per se*. The principle that a person has a claim against another due to whose negligence that person suffers need not be limited to cases of postnatal or even post-conception negligence. In *Renslow* v *Mennonite Hospital*.[79] liability was recognized for negligence which occurred over seven years before the plaintiff's conception.

A number of jurisdictions resist this conclusion, on the ground that duties cannot be owed to persons not conceived. This echoes earlier claims that duties cannot be owed to persons before they are born. When it is accepted, however, that civil law duties can be owed to third parties from special relationships, such as arise, for instance, between doctor and patient.[80] it is an unnecessary and often unjust limitation that those subsequently injured third parties must already have been born or conceived at the time of the breach of such duties. The defendant's power to limit liability should arise through a statute of limitation, not the chance date of the victim's birth.

The fallacy of foetal rights is at risk of extension as foetuses become medically treatable and are idealized and personified by advocates against abortion. Introductions to academic analyses that begin with such expressions as 'The expansion of foetal rights in tort law has prompted judicial consideration of . . .'[81] and literature titles such as 'The necessity of granting a cause of action to an unborn viable fetus . . .'[82] cause confusion. Similarly misguided is judicial reasoning which claims that, because the difference in biological status between a child of advanced gestation *in utero* and a newborn child is slight stillborn foetuses should have estates on behalf of which actions can be maintained as do born children.[83] Foetuses, as such, do not have legal rights. Born persons have legal rights which may arise for injuries caused, for instance, before they were born or before they were conceived. Similarly, they may claim on birth to receive bequests made in anticipation of their live birth. Those who have conceived but lost their foetuses due to another's negligence have, or should have, their own rights to sue. Their legal rights are separate, however, from any legal rights vested in the lost foetus *per se*. Persons so injured through legal negligence as to become sterile, and women so injured as to be incapable of conceiving or gestating children, pursue remedies when no foetus exists, and the same should be the case when a foetus comes into existence, however, briefly.

Accordingly, distinctions based on foetal viability are as arbitrary and irrelevant as advocates of foetal rights claim is the distinction between birth and full gestation before birth. A common paradigm of the argument for foetal rights is the case of identical twins. In a negligently caused accident, one is so injured that, following its live birth, it dies in hours. The other dies at full gestation, but before live birth. It is argued that it is unjust that a cause of action can be successful in the former case, but not in the latter. The next stage of reasoning is that no difference exists between a foetus of full gestational age and one which has reached viability, and that claims therefore should be allowed on the stillbirth of any viable foetus. The concluding step in this incremental regression is that, since viability is a medical criterion of unspecified content.[84] no distinction can be drawn between viable and pre-viable foetuses. Therefore, to avoid one arbitrary distinction replacing another (birth, full gestation or viability) it is urged that 'conception, therefore, should be the only prerequisite to finding a 'person' whose death is compensable under a wrongful death statute'.[85]

It is submitted that the criterion of conception is as arbitrary and irrelevant as any other. The goal of compensating those denied, through negligence, the desired experience of being parents of their genetic children should not distinguish those whose conceptions are caused to fail from those rendered unable to conceive. Those who fail to conceive and those whose conceptions fail should equally be able to sue for their losses, and be equally obliged to discharge the burden of proving on a balance of probability that, but for the negligence rendering them unable to conceive or have children, they would have become parents.

This burden is relatively easy to discharge regarding a foetus of full, or close to full, gestational age but becomes progressively harder to satisfy the earlier back one goes before the prospective birth, viability or conception of a foetus. About one in six, or even five, couples of reproductive age is infertile.[86] Evidence indicates that only about 22 per cent of fertilized ova are born alive.[87] and that about 62 per cent of pregnancies spontaneously abort in the first 12 weeks of gestation.[88] Those arguing that they are denied parenthood because they wrongly fail to conceive are thus little different from those arguing that their conceptions wrongly failed. The difference between them may concern only the quantum of damages representing their loss, including such heads of damage as suffering and discomfort in pregnancy and the experience of foetal loss or stillbirth.[89]

It should not be presumed that courts interpret their wrongful death legislation as being concerned only or at all with compensating plaintiffs for lost opportunities to be parents of their own children, and for injuries associated with failed pregnancy and stillbirth. Most US jurisdictions apply this presumption, but several enquire whether the legislature's intention was to protect the foetus itself. The Arizona Supreme Court, for instance, has consulted manslaughter and abortion legislation to determine whether the legislature protected foetuses themselves rather than their parents' interests in them.[90] Similarly, a Missouri court relied on the state's (later repealed) foeticide statute to find an intention to protect both decedents' survivors and foetuses themselves.[91] Alabama has considered its legislation to be punitive in intent, even though it provides for both compensatory and punitive damages.[92]

The issue of damages under wrongful death laws further shows how varied and confused are judicial approaches. The North Carolina Supreme Court has denied recovery for foetal loss under its statute, observing that ' . . . it can hardly be seriously contended that the death of a foetus represents *any* real pecuniary loss to the parents'.[93] This reflects an approach that parents' claims for their own injuries from incidents also causing foetal death will afford appropriate compensation, that claims are for only material or pecuniary losses, and that claims for foetal loss would present parents with windfall damages and double recovery. Claims for purely psychic injury have long been considered suspect, and, under the 'impact rule', were customarily dismissed where no physical injury had been suffered by the claimant.[94] Vagueness of claims for psychic suffering triggered judicial fears that such claims could be too easily feigned for the purpose of increasing the volume of recoverable damages.

Conservative courts have denied recovery for foetal loss on the pedantic grounds that 'person' in the jurisdictions' wrongful life statute conforms to the long-standing common law understanding of not including the unborn, and that the statute intends to cover the whole field of liability for wrongful death and leave the judiciary no residual capacity to expand the law.[95] Others have invoked policy reasons which, in contrast to those used to favour recovery, deny recovery on the basis that the legislature is not taken to intend recovery of highly speculative damages by parents.[96] As against this, however, courts in Massachusetts and Rhode Island for instance, have held that the nature of the damages and associated difficulties in assessment should not bar a right of action, and that mere difficulty of proof of damage or of causation should similarly not frustrate an action.[97] This is in contrast, of course, to much of the reasoning under which wrongful life claims by handicapped children continue to be dismissed.[98]

Courts more sympathetic to parental claims find that the purpose of wrongful death statutes is to compensate the parents not only for loss of the financial advantages children would represent to them, but for loss of companionship and well recognized parental satisfactions, and also for expenses associated with the incident of stillbirth. Courts have moved in this direction relatively strongly in recent years, compatibly with the movement away from suspicion of claims for psychic injuries and towards recognition that emotional distress and suffering alone can found a claim if provable by orthodox tort principles.[99] This modern approach merges statutory wrongful death claims with common law actions by parents for their own injuries from stillbirth, which now may include damages for emotional distress. Reading wrongful death statutes as being compatible with evolving common law principles which allow parents to claim for their own losses may do some violence, of course, to the origin of Lord Campbell's Act in *Baker* v. *Bolton*.[100] Some courts have considered this case to have been narrowly decided, however,[101] and that the 1846 Act may have enacted what the common law also allowed.

Momentum to advance stillborn foetal rights as such, rather than parental claims for their own injuries due to negligently inflicted foetal loss, comes from the perception that liability to pay compensation should be a deterrent to causing foetal loss. The Pro-Life preference is not served by parental compensation for loss since anti-abortion advocates consider parents to be a suspect class which endangers foetuses. Compensating parents leaves them free to cause foetal wastage. Such advocates accordingly employ and encourage reasoning that focuses on the lost foetus itself. This causes confusion in jurisprudence, however, and is open to question on ethical grounds in that it uses lost foetuses as an instrumental means to achieve the end of so promoting social perception of foetuses as to inhibit provision of abortion services.[102]

Foetal compensation is futile or misguided when the negligent or deliberate act which results in stillbirth is that of the parents. Where parents have legal rights to achieve abortion, of course, the loss or death of the foetus is not legally 'wrongful'. Doctrines of parental immunity for negligence, historically designed to maintain tranquillity of families by precluding divisive litigation, are now in decline in the USA.[103] Paradoxically, they never arose in the UK but now may be emerging under the Congenital Disabilities (Civil Liability) Act 1976.[104] Even when parents can be sued for negligence by their children, however, suit on behalf of lost foetuses raises the issue of what happens to awarded damages. If the parents inherit the estate, they recover their own money, which is futile except insofar as they are burdened with additional payments of legal costs. If they lose entitlement to succeed to the estate of the foetus, because in law they cannot profit from their own wrong,[105] and it passes to the Crown or sovereign as *bona vacantia*, the compensatory remedy becomes converted into a penalty or fine. As such, it should be levied only in accordance with the procedures and evidentiary standards of criminal process. Punitive damages are available to enhance the goals of civil compensation, but it is misguided that legislation enacted for civil compensation should be employed for an exclusively punitive purpose.

In this regard it is instructive to observe how wary US courts have been to hold that foetuses are intended to be covered in vehicular homicide legislation. Indeed, until the 1984 Massachusetts Supreme Judicial Court case of *Commonwealth v Cass*.[106] no US jurisdiction had included viable foetuses in a general definition of 'person' through judicial interpretation of a penal statute. Legislatures may have exercised power expressly to penalize deliberate or negligent foeticide, but objection has been taken to courts so interpreting existing legislation and reversing settled precedents in this novel way.[107]

An equally menacing use of criminal law was attempted in the October 1986 indictment in California of Pamela Rae Stewart (married name Monson) for failing to heed medical advice and to summon medical help for her child before birth.[108] The criminal charge was dismissed when the judge rejected the prosecutor's contention of legislative intent,[109] but the incident confirms how foetal protection has become an instrument used against parents, particularly mothers.

In recent years, courts in the USA have considered it appropriate to protect viable foetuses by ordering that pregnant women be exposed to medical treatment over their objections, even to the extent of authorizing non-consensual surgery as invasive as ceasarean delivery.[110] The creation of foetal rights has evolved to present a fundamental challenge to women's autonomy, and to reverse the welcome trend of recent decades towards recognition of women's entitlements to receive respect and equal treatment. The newer development renders women subordinate to the interests of perceived others – namely their foetuses.[111] It may appear ironic that the Pro-Life concern with foetuses results in women's interests being placed in opposition to their unborn children's interests, to the detriment of the family unit, when Pro-Life advocates often maintain as an alternative, that they are Pro-Family. This development exposes the reactionary character of the Pro-Life philosophy as favouring a situation where pregnant women are liable to coercive legal constraints and are considered untrustworthy to make decisions in the best interests of their families. It confirms a maledominated vision that the most important facet of a woman is her reproductive role, through which she is controllable.[112]

The liability of health professionals and health facilities to be ordered to pay compensation to the estate of a foetus for its wrongful death provides them with an incentive to take legal action against pregnant women. Medical advice to a pregnant patient is thereby converted into a legally enforceable order that she obey medical instructions, and health professionals are thereby transformed from helpers to gaolers who possess legal power to detain her, render her unconscious if they wish, and cut open her abdomen in order to serve the primary object of legal protection, the foetus.

It is acknowledged that '[A]mong the most harrowing experiences for obstetricians is the refusal of therapy by a pregnant woman'.[113] However, requests for court-ordered interventions against women may not afford a solution for health professionals or, indeed, for foetuses. Legal powers recognized to reside in health practitioners to invoke the courts' authority in order to usurp patients' decision-making rights on behalf of foetuses and their families can easily be legally transformed into legal duties. Health practitioners who decline to invoke such power may become liable to suit on behalf of the foetuses they failed to act to save. Legal duties have been recognized which oblige mental health practitioners in particular to take action against their patients' wishes in order to protect third parties they perceive, or competently should perceive, to be threatened by the patients.[114] Such duties may be more acutely binding on obstetricians, since they have developed concepts and rhetoric that recognize foetuses as being patients separate from the mothers who bear them. The forging of legal links of responsibility to such foetal patients could be founded on existing legal doctrine, and reinforced by the obligations which obstetricians and related health professionals claim to have assumed.

The risk this presents to foetuses is apparent in the USA in the growing scarcity of doctors specializing in prenatal care and obstetrics. Increasing legal liabilities which courts have found for injuries suffered by newborn children due to inadequate foetal monitoring and other deficiencies in prenatal care have been related to health professionals disfavouring and abandoning these special-ities, and to the emergence of midwives and paramedical personnel to provide birth management services. Physicians believe that this trend compromises the standard of medical care for the unborn. This result may not be aggravated by an increasing risk of legal suit on behalf of stillborn foetuses, however, since a factor influencing the US development has been the large damage awards given to injured children who face a lifetime of costly medical treatment and nursing services due to negligent prenatal care – a situation which does not apply to stillborn foetuses. Damages awarded to estates of the stillborn might include a punitive element, however, since activist courts, anxious to protect foetuses as such, might be reluc-tant to compromise protection by awards of trivial or inconsequen-tial damages.

Wrongful death claims on behalf of stillborn foetuses *per se* have not been allowed or judicially considered in any detail in such jurisdictions as the UK, Australia and Canada. It is argued and urged here that they should not be. On the other hand, it is contended that the general law or wrongful death statutes should be read to provide compensation for those whose reasonable ambitions to be parents are wrongfully frustrated due to others' negligence which results in foetal loss. Awards through which would-be parents recover compensation for medical and related costs, for pain, and for their emotional distress should follow prevailing principles of assessment in injury cases. Such awards are no more likely to deter health professionals from rendering care than awards made in other medical cases, and would fall far below the enormity of sums needed to maintain seriously handicapped newborns for decades of costly medical and nursing care.

The capacity of courts to recognize and compensate parental damages for the wrongful death of a foetus predates the movement towards separate recognition of the foetus itself. In 1969, for instance, the New York Court of Appeals allowed damages when a foetus was killed *in utero* in order to compensate the mother for her physical and mental injuries, including the emotional trauma of the stillbirth.[115] The father also recovered for loss of his wife's services and loss of consortium. With the decline of the 'impact rule', which limited recovery for psychic harm when no physical contact or effect was provable, damages would also be recoverable for his proven distress from the stillbirth. Courts and legislatures increasingly permit parents to recover for the loss of comfort, society and companionship of a child. The New York court added, however, that:

> . . . additional award to the distributees' of the foetus would give its parents an unmerited bounty and would constitute not compensation to the injured but punishment to the wrongdoer.[116]

This limitation reveals a clarity of principle which later decisions have sacrificed in their misguided attempts to give protection to future foetuses and 'compensation' to those which have been lost before live birth.

Claims brought under wrongful death statutes on behalf of still-born foetuses are unnecessary where the general law permits parents to recover in their own right for their injuries resulting from negligent infliction of foetal loss. In England, the Queen's Bench Division heard such a claim for recovery in mid-1986.[117] A hospital admitted its liability for negligently failing to conduct blood analysis on a patient known to have blood incompatibility with her foetus, and for failing to offer early surgical delivery of the child, resulting in stillbirth. The only issue before the court was the quantum of general damages, and the approach taken gives some guidance on how such claims are currently resolved. The fact that liability was admitted is significant, not just of the defendant's candid approach to the facts but of its legally-advised approach to the credibility of the legal claim. Public bodies such as health authorities cannot concede legal claims and agree to settle them from public funds unless they have legal substance. The case demonstrates not simply the principles of assessment of general damages, but also an important principle of legal liability under generally prevailing law. The action invoked no contorted or contrived claim on behalf of a foetus or its estate under the Fatal Accidents Act 1846.

Consistently with prevailing law, the judge excluded from the claim for general damages any item for grief and sorrow.[118] Whilst refusal to compensate disappointment is understandable on grounds of vagueness, US courts increasingly admit heads of damage for outrage when psychic injury is deliberately caused, and for negligent infliction of emotional distress. It is submitted that this trend is sound and just in principle, although perhaps only modest amounts should be awarded except in clear cases of foresee-able, and therefore preventable, injury. The Administration of Justice Act 1982 made bereavement recoverable under the Fatal Accidents Act 1846 in the fixed sum of £3,500, but only on loss of a born person. The court could not therefore make a direct award for bereavement on foetal loss. This again seems harsh where a foetus is of such advanced gestational age that the experience of its society is likely and imminent. The unborn can be experienced only in concept, whereas the born are more personally knowable to the senses, but this in itself may justify modest damages for loss of reasonable expectation of future society of lost foetuses rather than total exclusion of parents' claims. A more compassionate approach to the issue is realistic, and may require legislative reconsideration of eligibility for compensation for bereavement.

The judge found three interacting heads of damage, namely:

(i) loss of satisfaction of bringing pregnancy (and, in this case, confinement and labour) to a successful conclusion;

(ii) loss associated with physical loss of the child, notably frustration of plans to found or enlarge a family; and

(iii) physical illness and suffering directly experienced by the plaintiff due to the proven negligence.

The judge found analogies between the items covered by heads (i) and (ii) and the claim for bereavement recoverable for death of a child. This approach reduces the need for legislative reconsideration of statutory limitations on compensation for bereavement. The judge also found an analogy under head (ii) between foetal loss and loss of the society of a born child, finding that little real distinction can be made between loss of rearing a known newborn child and loss of rearing an advanced foetus which could have lived but which, through negligence, was stillborn. Aggregating entitlements under the three recognized heads of claim, the judge found that the sum of £18,000 was appropriate as general damages.

Awards to plaintiffs denied wanted parenthood assessed according to these realistic heads of legal damage do justice to claims for compensation for negligent infliction of foetal loss. The foetus itself or its estate is not an appropriate claimant, however, and arguments contending that a stillborn foetus should be recognized as a plaintiff confuse, distort and abuse prevailing juisprudence.

Conclusion

Sensitivity to the time lag between medical advances and their accommodation in law may induce legal commentators and judges to embrace new medical perceptions with uncritical enthusiasm. An excitement with technology may similarly induce ill-considered acceptance in law of biomedical imperatives – such as recognition of foetuses as patients distinct from their mothers. Against this, however, fear or suspicion of novelty in medical techniques or human relationships arising through such techniques can cause the law to implode around inert concepts, and to sacrifice its elasticity and tolerance to change. Reactions to biomedical developments in such fields as both containment and promotion of human reproduction, prenatal diagnosis and neonatology have ranged from blurring important legal distinctions between actual and potential bearers of rights and duties to moral panic lest new medical visions and possibilities may expose inadequacies in legal concepts, such as parenthood and the family.

Legal claims for wrongful birth, wrongful life and wrongful causing of stillbirth or death before birth have disclosed judicial responses of reactionary insistence that human birth is a benefit which transcends all detriments and that, for instance, legislatures can be taken to have intended to compensate lost foetuses separately from their parents. Improbable though such findings may be to lay observers, they have been seized, particularly by Pro-Life activists, in order to manipulate jurisprudence to serve their agenda. Items on this agenda include isolation and independent promotion of claims on behalf of foetuses, and denial of legal remedies to parents and children who appear unwelcoming of the 'gift' of human life because it is grossly handicapped. A consistent item is the reduction of women's autonomy in the medical management of their pregnancies, and of parents' control of the composition of their families.

It is argued here that the law retains its integrity and potential to achieve justice in society by advancing living claimants' ability to receive compensation for their experiences of pain, distress and financial costs which are attributable to others' deliberate or negligent failure to prevent such predictable harms. This should be so whether such failure occurs when they are living, unborn or not yet conceived. Further, it is argued that legal personhood should not be recognized in foetuses as such, but that the general proposition to be maintained that live birth is the precondition to admission of legal claims. Negligent infliction of foetal loss – as of death to living human beings – should afford rights to born claimants, but not to the stillborn or dead.

An incongruity of Pro-Life reasoning is that it argues for wrongful death claims for foetuses on the ground that there is no difference between a child born alive and a viable foetus *in utero*. It is contended that, since the former can claim for injuries causing death, justice requires that the latter should also be able to claim. It may equally be argued, however, that if a foetus has a right of action when it suffers stillbirth *in utero*, a handicapped newborn child should, in justice, also have a cause of action for pain and suffering. Pro-Life advocates oppose the claims of such children, however, overreacting perhaps to the term 'wrongful life' but motivated primarily by fear that doctors will seek to evade liability to them through abortion. This disregards the possibility, however, that parents who know that compensation will be unavailable from those due to whose negligence their handcapped children are born will seek abortions.

This confirms the inadequacy of a policy of developing tort law in order to affect the incidence of abortion. Attempts to refashion tort law judicially or by statute so that it may serve as a weapon in the abortion conflict will lead to distortion and corruption of the law, and should be resisted. Tort law should continue to evolve according to its historic function of providing for the compensation of those members of society who experience pain, suffering, distress or loss due to the negligence of others who owe them a duty to exercise care.

Notes

1 For convenience, reference will generally be made to the law of tort as if it were synonymous with the law of delict although it is acknowledged that the two have different histories and traditions. Only where the two systems produce notably different results will the distinction be expressly noted.

2 Maternal mortality is defined as the death of a woman who is pregnant or has been pregnant within 42 days prior to death; see World Health Organization, *Prevention of Maternal Mortality*, Geneva, WHO, 1985, p. 5.

3 Language has assumed particular symbolism in the context of abortion. The expression 'foetus' will be used here to describe an unborn human, although at times it includes what biologists might call an embryo or earlier form of human life, and what others might describe as an unborn child.

4 See Dickens, B. M., 'Abortion, amniocentesis and the law' 34 *American Journal of Comparative Law*, 1986, 249.

5 Classically, a 'human being' is one born alive, following complete removal from the mother's body, whether or not the child has breathed or has a separate circulation, or the umbilical cord is severed. With development of foetal treatment *extra uterum*, policy suggests that the concept of birth should mean permanent evacuation from the mother's womb, and not brief, temporary removal; see Dickens, *loc. cit.*, note 4 *supra*, pp. 219–21.

6 For further discussion of the abortion debate, see Chapter 3, *supra*.

7 See generally Special Project, 'Legal rights and issues surrounding conception, pregnancy, and birth', **39** *Vanderbilt Law Review*, 1986, 597. 724 *et seq.*

8 None of these claims has resulted in an award of damages in the US; see *Zapeda* v. *Zapeda* (1963), 190 N.E. 2d 849 (111.CA). The issue is not discussed hereafter, but is raised simply because the Zapeda judgement spoke of this early case as being for wrongful birth.

9 See *Udale* v. *Bloomsbury Area Health Authority* [1981] 2 All ER 522 (QBD) at p. 531.

10 *Troppi* v. *Scarf* (1971), 187 NW 2d 511 (Mich. CA) at p. 517. This language and reasoning were echoed by Mr Justice Pain in *Thake* v. *Maurice*, [1984] 2 All ER 513 (QBD) at p. 526.
11 See note 7, *supra*, p. 732.
12 *Emeh* v. *Kensington and Chelsea and Westminster Area Health Authority*, [1984] 3 All ER 1044 (CA), and *Thake* v. *Maurice*, [1986] 1 All ER 497 (CA).
13 The legality of sterilization was recognized in the English Court of Appeal in, for instance, *Bravery* v. *Bravery* [1954] 3 All ER 59.
14 *Gleitman* v. *Cosgrove* (1967), 227 A. 2d 689 (NJSC).
15 Note 14, *supra*, at p. 693.
16 Ibid., at p. 703, *per* Justice Jacobs
17 *Roe* v. *Wade* (1973), 410 US 113; *Doe* v. *Bolton* (1973), 410 US 179.
18 Smith, D. C., 'Wrongful birth, wrongful life: emerging theories of liability' in Butler, J. D. and Walbert, F. (eds.), *Abortion, Medicine and the Law*, 3rd. edn., 1986, 178 at p. 181.
19 *Watt* v. *Rama*, [1972] VR 353 (Vic. SC).
20 See *McKay* v. *Essex Area Health Authority*, [1982] 1 QB 1161 (CA).
21 See, for example, the damage award exceeding $1 million, reduced on appeal because of the availability of public health insurance services, in *Wipfli* v. *Britten* (1984), 13 DLR (4th) 169 (Brit. Col. CA).
22 *Zimmer* v. *Ringrose*, (1981), 124 DLR (3d) 215 (Alta. CA)
23 In New Zealand, common law actions for damages for personal injury were abolished by the Accident Compensation Act 1972, s. 5(1) (now consolidated by the Accident Compensation Act 1982). For a critique of the relevant New Zealand position on this topic now, see O'Neill, C. J., 'Damages and the unwanted child' 5 *Auckland University Law Review*, 180, 1985, at 198–205.
24 See the appeal decision, note 12, *supra*.
25 See *The Times*, 3 March 1983. Law Reports, High Court, discussed in the Court of Appeal, note 12, *supra*.
26 See note 12, *supra*, at p. 1048.
27 Ibid., at p. 1053.
28 *Troppi* v. *Scarf*, note 10, *supra*., at p. 520.
29 See text and reference at note 11 *supra*.
30 The child's own right to recover for loss of expectation of life raises issues relevant to the wrongful life action, considered below. The claim for the child's loss of expectation of life is itself incongruent with a parent's claim that the child should not have been conceived or born. Further, if its life is painful to the child, the fact that the life is of lesser duration than normal may be a mitigating, rather than an aggravating, factor.
31 *Doiron* v. *Orr*, (1978), 86 DLR (3d) 719 (Ont. High Ct.)
32 Ibid., pp. 722–3.
33 *Cataford* v. *Moreau* (1978), 114 DLR (3d) 585 (Que Superior Ct.).
34 Note 10, *supra*.
35 1d.
36 Bickenbach, J. E., 'Damages for wrongful conception: *Doiron* v. *Orr*', **18** U. *Western Ontario Law Review*, 1980, 493, at 498.
37 See Goldstein, J., Freud, A., and Solnit, A., *Beyond the Best Interests of the Child*, new edn., New York, The Free Press, 1979.
38 See note 32, *supra*.
39 *Merritt* v. *Parker* 1 NJL 526 (NJ 1795).
40 See note 20, *supra*.
41 See note 9, *supra*.
42 Law Commission of England and Wales, *Report on Injuries to Unborn Children*, 1974 Law Com. no. 69, Cmnd. 5709, para 89, p. 34.

43 1d.
44 *Sidaway* v. *Board of Governors of the Bethlem Royal Hospital and the Maudsley Hospital*, [1985] 1 AC 871 (HL)
45 *Reibl* v. *Hughes* (1980), 114 DLR (3d) 1, adopting *Canterbury* v. *Spence* (1972), 464 F. 2d 772 and *Cobbs* v. *Grant* (1972), 104 Cal. Rptr. 505.
46 Minn. Stat. Ann. Section 145.424; Missouri Stat. Ann. Section 188.130; Utah Stat. Ann. Section 76.7 – 305.5.
47 *Hickman* v. *Group Health Plan, Inc.* (1986), 396 NW 2d 10 (Minn. SC)
48 *Bowen* v. *American Hospital Association* 106 S.Ct. 2101 (1986).
49 See Special Project, note 7, *supra* at pp. 752–5.
50 Note 14, *supra*.
51 *Procanik* v. *Cillo* (1984), 478 A. 2d 755 (NJSC).
52 In addition to the three in note 46, *supra*, California and, for instance, South Dakota have legislated against the action, and there is pressure in several other states: see Cal. Civil Code Section 43.6, and SD Cod. L. Ann Sections 21–55 (1981).
53 Note 14, *supra*, p. 692.
54 See note 17, *supra*.
55 See, for example, Pace, D. H., 'The treatment of injury in wrongful life claims', **20**, *Columbia Journal of Law and Social Problems*, 1986, 145.
56 See note 42, *supra*.
57 In allowing the wrongful life action, the New Jersey Supreme Court in *Procanik* v. *Cillo* observed that 'Law is more than an exercise in logic, and logical analysis, although essential to a system of ordered justice, should not become an instrument of injustice'; note 51, *supra*, at p. 762.
58 See Ranous, J. S. and Sherrin, J. J., 'Busting the blessing balloon: liability for the birth of an unplanned child', **39** *Albany Law Review*, 1975, 221.
59 *Continental Casualty Co.* v. *Empire Casualty Co.*, No. 83CAD 139 (Colorado Ct. Appl. 27 June 1985), quoted in Special Project, note 7 *supra*, p. 765.
60 *Supra cit.*
61 *In the Matter of Karen Quinlan* (1976), 355 A. 2d 647 (NJSC).
62 See the discussion in *Tarasoff* v. *Regents of the University of California* (1976), 551 P. 2d 334 (Cal. SC).
63 See, generally, *Renslow* v. *Mennonite Hospital* (1977), 367 NE 2d 1250 (Ill. SC).
64 See, for example, *Becker* v. *Schwartz* (1978), 386 NE 2d 807 (NYCA).
65 *Harbeson* v. *Parke-Davis* (1983), 656 P. 2d 483 (Wash. SC)
66 See note 20, *supra*.
67 See note 42, *supra*.
68 Indeed, it may be contended that, as parents, they are legally entitled and obliged to make the decision on behalf of the child: see Handler J. in *Procanik* v. *Cillo*, note 51, *supra*. at p. 769. In *Curlender* v. *Bio-Science Laboratories* (1980), 106 Cal. App. 3d 811, the court approving a wrongful life action said, *obiter*, that it might be brought against a parent, but this observation is generally considered to be unsound.
69 Cf. Mason, J. K. and McCall Smith, R. A., *Law and Medical Ethics*, 2nd edn., London, Butterworths, 1987, p. 99 n. 17.
70 On different approaches taken to damages where wrongful life claims have been allowed, see Special Project, note 7 *supra*, p. 767.
71 See Special Project, note 7 *supra*, p. 782.
72 *Baker* v. *Bolton* (1808), 170 Eng. Rep. 1033 (KB).
73 9 & 10 Vict., ch. 93.
74 See Starczewski, M., 'Note: wrongful death of a fetus: does a cause of action arise when there is no live birth?' **31** *Villanova Law Review*, 1986, 669. at p. 683.

75 See, for example, Keyserlingk, E. W., *The Unborn Child's Rights to Prenatal Care: A Comparative Law Perspective* McGill Legal Studies no. 5, Montreal, Quebec Research Centre of Private and Comparative Law, 1984.

76 See note 5, *supra*.

77 See the influential Massachusetts Supreme Court case *Dietrich* v. *Northampton* (1984), 138 Mass. 14.

78 *Bonbrest* v. *Kotz* (1946), 65 F. Supp. 138 (US Dist. Ct. for Dist. of Columbia).

79 Note 63, *supra*.

80 See, for example, the fiduciary and tortious duties recognized in *Tarasoff* v. *Regents of the University of California*, note 62 supra.

81 See Special Project, note 7, *supra*., at p. 771.

82 See, for example, McClelland, R. M., 'The necessity of granting a cause of action to an unborn viable fetus under the Pennsylvania wrongful death and survival acts'. **21** *Duquesne Law Review*, 1983, 1017.

83 See, for example, *Amadio* v. *Levin* (1985) 501 A. 2d 1085 (Pa. SC).

84 'Viability' does not distinguish between independent and dependent viability. Prematurely born children are viable at increasingly early stages of gestation because of mechanical life-supports. Further, embryos may be viable for some time *in vitro* before implantation in a woman's uterus.

85 See Special Project, note 7, *supra*, p. 786.

86 See Hull, M. G. R., 'Infertility: nature and extent of the problem' in the CIBA Foundation, *Human Embryo Research: Yes or No?*, London Tavistock, 1986, p. 24. Infertility is commonly defined as inability to conceive by normal sexual intercourse after two years of trying but, if the definition is taken as non-conception in one year of trying, the incidence is greater.

87 Roberts, C. J. and Lowe, D. B., 'Where have all the conceptions gone?', *Lancet* no. 1 1975, p. 498.

88 Edmonds, D. K., Lindsay, K. S., *et al.*, 'Early embryonic mortality in women', **38** (4) *Fertility and Sterility*, 1982, 447; on legal implications of this, see Cook, R. J., 'Legal abortion: limits and contributions to human life' in CIBA Foundation Symposium 115, *Abortion: Medical Progress and Social Implications*, London, Pitman, 1985, p. 24.

89 Stillbirth is conventionally defined as delivery of a dead foetus that has completed 20 weeks' gestation. Statutes or regulations often require the delivery of a dead foetus after 20 weeks' gestation, or one which weighs 500 grams, to be registered as stillbirth.

90 *Summerfield* v. *Superior Court* (1985), 698 p. 2d 712 (en banc).

91 *O'Grady* v. *Brown* (1983), 654 SW 2d 904. (en banc).

92 *Eich* v. *town of Gulf Shores* (1974), 300 So. 2d 354 (Ala SC).

93 *Gay* v. *Thompson* (1966), 146 SE 2d 425. at p. 428.

94 See Bell, P. A., 'The bell tolls: toward full tort recovery for psychic injury', **36** *University of Florida Law Review*, 1984, 333.

95 See, for instance, the California Supreme Court in *Justus* v. *Atchinson* (1977), 565 P. 2d 122 (en banc).

96 See the New Jersey Supreme Court in *Grav* v. *Taggert* (1964), 204 A. 2d 140 and the New York Court of Appeals in *Endresz* v. *Friedberg* (1969), 248 NE 2d 901.

97 See, respectively, *Mone* v. *Greyhound Lines, Inc.* (1975), 331 NE 2d 916 and *Presley* v. *Newport Hospital* (1976), 365 A. 2d 748.

98 See text above, at note 53.

99 See Bell, loc. cit., note 94 *supra*.

100 See note 72, *supra*.

101 See the Arizona Supreme Court in *Summerfield* v. *Superior Court*, note 90, *supra* at p. 716.

102   See Callahan, D., 'How technology is reframing the abortion debate'. **16**(1) *Hastings Center Report*, 1988, 33.
103   See, for example, *Gelbman* v. *Gelbman* (1969), 245 NE 2d 192, abolishing intrafamilial tort immunity in the state of New York.
104   This applies only to England and Wales. The Report of the Scottish Law Commission, *Liability for Ante-Natal Injury*, Cmnd. 5371, 1973, which did not result in legislation in Scotland, left the pre-existing common law position intact – namely that children could sue either parent.
105   See Youfan, T. G., 'Acquisition of property by killing', **89** *Law Quarterly Review*, 1973, 235.
106   *Commonwealth* v. *Cass*, (1984), 467 N.E. 2d 1324.
107   See Palmer, B., 'State protection of future "persons": *Commonwealth* v. *Cass*'. **18** *Connecticut Law Review*, 1986, 429.
108   See Balisy, S. S., 'Maternal substance abuse: the need to provide protection for the fetus', **60** *Southern California Law Review*, 1987, 1209.
109   See *New York Times*, 28 February 1987, p. 32.
110   See, for example, *Jefferson* v. *Griffin Spalding County Hospital Authority* (1981). 274 SE 2d 457 (Georgia SC) and, generally, Kolder, V. E. B., Gallagher, J. and Parsons, M. T., 'Court-ordered obstetrical interventions'. **317** *New England Journal of Medicine*, 1987, 1192, reporting at least eleven US states that have ordered caesarian deliveries.
111   See Johnsen, D. E., 'The creation of fetal rights: conflicts with Women's constitutional rights to liberty, privacy, and equal protection'. **95** *Yale Law Journal*, 1986, 599.
112   See Annas, G. J., 'Pregnant women as fetal containers', **16**(6) *Hastings Center Report*, 1986, 13.
113   Kolder *et. al*, p. 1194.
114   See the Tarasoff case, note 62, *supra*.
115   *Endresz* v. *Friedberg*, note 96, *supra*. In Scottish Law, the death of a foetus *in utero* which is caused by another's negligence was accepted as a potential element in an action for damages raised by the mother – *Bourhill* v. *Young* 1941 SC 395, esp. p. 431.
116   *Endresz* note 96, *supra*, p. 904.
117   '*Bagley* v. *North Herts Health Authority* (30 July 1986, Simon Brown J., QBD)', **136** *Law Journal*, 1986, 1014.
118   Following *McLaughlin* v. *O'Brien* [1982] 2 All ER 289, *per* Lord Wilberforce, pp. 301–2.

5 Selective non-treatment of handicapped infants

DAVID MEYERS

Introduction

Advances in neonatology have permitted significant improvement in infant survival rates, and newborns can now be sustained with multiple defects which would have previously proven fatal. Approximately 7 per cent of live births produce abnormal infants. Each year in America some 40,000 infants are born with birthweights of less than 1,500 grammes,[1] and their care will often involve life and death decisions as to whether all treatments available should be pursued.

These cases pose medical, legal and ethical dilemmas in respect of treatment. What is treatment? Is it provision of food and water? How intensive or invasive should treatment be when its life-prolongation or life-enhancement benefit is limited? Should treatment ever be withheld? If so, in what instances and why? Who should decide these questions? What role do the parents play? What role do the physicians play? Who speaks for the interests of the infant? What would the infant want done and who, in certain cases, can possibly know or presume to know? Who can say that withholding or withdrawing treatment from a handicapped infant is ever in his or her 'best interests'?

There are many questions to answer. More questions than we have answers. But they are important and need and deserve answers, and those that have so far been offered are, in large part, tentative and arguably ambiguous. This is, however, an area of human concern that abounds with ambiguity. The condition of one infant represents differences – at times only subtle shadings of differences – from that of another. Physicians' and parents' judgements are just that. They are hopefully informed, but inevitably

113

subjective, and undoubtedly reflective of bias, background and situation.

However, as in most human endeavour, what is sought here is fairness, not perfection. Little abuse seems to have flowed from the attitude to benign neglect which has prevented, in very large part, formalization of decision-making or its review in this area. The outlines of some principles, some standards of conduct, and of judicial review, have begun to emerge. But, as will be seen, selective non-treatment of handicapped infants occurs against a backdrop of uncertain and, at times, inconsistent, medical practice and legal responsibility. Much is still to be considered, articulated and clarified on the road to medical, legal and ethical consensus.

Contemporary medical practice

There are numerous causes for significant handicaps in newborn infants. Perhaps the most prevalent cause is infants born below average birthweight because of prematurity. Low birthweights can result in a number of lifelong disabilities or complications for the infant, including respiratory insufficiency, brain injury or haemorrhage and other organ system dysfunction or disability.

Neural tube defects, from brain to tip of spine, can cause a substantial number of birth handicaps. When a child is born suffering from anencephaly, most or all of the brain is missing. Hydranencephaly is a condition where most of the brain has failed to develop in the infant. Encephaloceles is a condition where the skull has not properly closed, allowing brain tissue to protrude. Finally, spina bifida is a condition where, because of abnormalities in the development of the spinal cord, a sack of nerve tissue protudes from the back. The site of the lesion in the spinal column can make a considerable difference in the disabilities expected from the handicap. Often, the infant is paralysed below the site of the lesion, suffers incontinence, neurological deficits and other problems. Patients born suffering from spina bifida systica have a premature mortality rate of more than fifty per cent.

Down's syndrome is a chromosomal abnormality that occurs in approximately every 600 to 700 live births in the USA.[2] It can cause mental retardation of various degrees, abnormalities of the hand, foot, eyelids and/or lip, reproductive disorders, congenital heart and gastrointestinal abnormalities and decreased muscle tone. However, it is generally recognized that the ability to predict the degree of mental retardation is poor in the early stages of infancy.

Until, approximately, the last 30 years, it was accepted medical practice not aggressively to treat such handicapped infants against the wishes of their parents. They generally were left at home or in institutions where most of them died during their infancy.[3]

However, more recently, with improved medical technology and greater understanding of these conditions, the medical community has taken more aggressive steps to treat such handicapped infants. Still, the debate continues in the medical profession as to when only nursing or comfort care should be given in such cases because of the futility of aggressive treatment in allowing for the infant's long-term survival without what is perceived to be an intolerable level of pain or disability.

Little was publicly known or written of concerning selective non-treatment of severely handicapped newborns until the early 1970s. In 1973 a pioneering article by two physicians – one American, one Scottish – was published, which discussed their practice and experience with such cases in a Northeast US neonatal clinic.[4] The doctors contended that their experience showed that the law should give substantial discretion to parents in authorizing or refusing to authorize active treatment for their severely deformed newborn. Precise guidelines were difficult to apply.

The law has lent a certain amount of support to this practice, given the deeply rooted principle of parental control over their infants.[5] Further, since young children are incapable of making intelligent decisions concerning their own well-being, parental consent is legally necessary before medical treatment may be undertaken – at least, in the absence of emergency.[6]

Parents have relied upon various humanitarian motives to withhold treatment for their handicapped infants. Some believe treatment is not in accord with their religious tenets. Some are concerned about the infant's 'quality of life', the burdens of the infant's continued life on others in the family, the pain of the proposed treatment, the limited benefit of the treatment in terms of extended life expectancy and, perhaps most importantly, the futility of the treatment.[7] Few cases of abuse have been reported.

The issue: quality of life

It is one thing to make quality of life judgements for an individual who has made his or her own wishes known on the subject, either because he or she is competent, or has expressed such wishes while they were competent. It is quite another consideration to attempt any evaluation of another's quality of life – as in the case of an infant – when that person has never expressed him or herself nor been capable of expressing him or herself on that subject. It must be asked whether a reasonable judgement on the quality of life of a severely handicapped infant can be made by a physically normal individual. Whilst a healthy individual may think that the quality of life of a severely handicapped infant would not make continued life worth living, surely that person cannot presume to speak for the handicapped infant him or herself, who may be, and very likely is, happy to be alive.

American courts, when asked to award a handicapped infant general damages for pain and suffering based on wrongful life, have refused. How can anyone say, most have reasoned, that the impaired life of a handicapped infant is worse for that child than the child never having been born at all? If one accepts that principle, which it seems exceedingly hard to refute or challenge, then it becomes extremely difficult to justify ever saying that it is in the best interests of an infant not to provide life-sustaining treatment because of handicap or defect. As one court has stated:

> Whether it is better never to have been born at all than to have been born with even gross deficiencies is a mystery more properly to be left to philosophers and the theologians. Surely the law can assert no competence to resolve the issue, particularly in view of the very nearly uniform high value which the law and mankind has placed on human life, rather than its absence. Not only is there to be found no predicate at common law or in statutory enactment for judicial recognition of the birth of a defective child as an injury to the child; the implications of any such proposition are staggering. Would claims be honored, assuming the breach of an identifiable duty, for less than a perfect birth? And by what standard or by whom would perfection be defined? There is also a second flaw. The remedy afforded an injured party in negligence is designed to place that party in the position he would have occupied but for the negligence of the defendant. Thus, the damages recoverable on behalf of an infant for wrongful life are limited to that which is necessary to restore the infant to the position he or she would have occupied were it not for the failure of the defendant to render advice to the infant's parents in a nonnegligent manner. The theoretical hurdle to an assertion of damages on behalf of an infant accruing from a defendant's negligence in such a case becomes at once apparent. The very allegations of the complaint state that had the defendant not been negligent, the infant's parent would have chosen not to conceive, or having conceived, to have terminated rather than to have carried the pregnancy to term, thereby depriving the infant plaintiff of his or her very existence. Simply put, a cause of action brought on behalf of an infant seeking recovery for wrongful life demands a calculation of damages dependent upon a comparison between the Hobson's choice of life in an impaired state and nonexistence. This comparison the law is not equipped to make.[8]

It seems that, so long as pain and discomfort are not overwhelming or intolerable, an infant's condition cannot be said to make it in its 'best interests' to have life-sustaining treatment withheld or withdrawn.[9] However, it may be proper to honour the parents' wishes and to elect against the imposition of finite medical resources where no conscious or interactional existence, no cognitive appreciation of life, will result for the infant.

In newborn non-treatment cases should not considerations of quality of life be limited to more objective phenomena of lack of cognition (here taken to mean the process of knowing, including awareness and judgement), or severe pain and physical discomfort? Judgement may be ventured when the physical pain and discomfort of a particular condition, or a treatment to alleviate it, are so severe and unremitting as to be 'inhumane' – something which no person could be expected physically to endure. In such circumstances it may be appropriate to withhold life-sustaining treatment where the prospect of continued life carries with it the continuation of severe, unremitting pain of such a degree as to rob the individual of the capability of the physical enjoyment of existence. In such situations, it may be better to concentrate on providing a shortened period of life, with tolerable pain, rather than an extension of that life with intolerable pain. However, quality of life in such situations is to be judged by physiological (taken to mean the characteristics of an individual's healthy or normal functioning) existence, rather than any concepts of social utility, intellectual capability or emotional happiness.

As one author has cogently stated:

> In sum, opinions regarding the value of life are so disparate, and ability to calculate an infant's capacity to enjoy life so feeble, that withholding treatment on the basis of the 'quality of life' rests life and death decisions on pure speculation.[10]

This criticism would seem not well taken where the infant is without the cognition to relate to other people and his or her environment. Here the basic characteristic of human existence and value is missing. But what have the courts said when confronted with such issues?

US legal precedent

Action by the Supreme Court

What must be remembered when considering how few infant non-treatment cases have reached the courts is that US law gives substantial weight and respect to parents' decisions concerning the medical treatment or non-treatment of their infant children. The US Supreme Court has rarely been called upon to act in this arena. However, in three recent cases it has reaffirmed, in broad outline and largely by implication, the wide degree of parental discretion that will be judicially accepted in such instances.

In the most recent of the cases, regulations promulgated by the Executive Branch of Government in the person of the Secretary of Health and Human Services were at issue. Under the authority of a statute[11] prohibiting discrimination on the basis of physical handicap in the implementation of any programme or activity receiving federal government financial assistance, the Secretary drew up comprehensive rules relating to proper health care for handicapped infants.[12] These included the required posting of informational notices in newborn nurseries, expedited federal review of medical records in cases of alleged medical neglect in the treatment of handicapped newborn, and the availability of a government 'hotline' to report by telephone any such alleged instances. Among the several examples of improper medical treatment referenced in the rules was the decision not to correct intestinal atresia (blockage due to incomplete formation) or oesophageal atresia in a Down's syndrome child, in the absence of the presence of a further physical complication medically warranting such inaction. While not addressing the relevance of parental non-consent to treatment in such a case, the implication of the rules was that it was irrelevant and that treatment must be provided. The examples did, however, acknowledge that there was no obligation to undertake 'futile treatment', such as in cases of anencephaly (lack of brain) or severe prematurity and low birthweight where treatment could 'do no more than temporarily prolong the act of dying'.

These rules were challenged by a group of medical organizations and physicians as improper and not statutorily authorized.

The interim rules had earlier been struck down as invalid by the second-circuit Federal Court of Appeals in New York.[13] Rather than seeking *certiorari* (review) in that case, the government amended its Final Rules, which were again challenged. On hearing, the US Supreme Court invalidated the rules as being beyond the authority conferred upon the Secretary by the Congress.[14]

In handing down its ruling, the US Supreme Court reiterated the principle that the law ' . . . vests decisional responsibility [for medical treatment of infants] in the parents, in the first instances, subject to review in exceptional cases by the State acting as parens patriae.'[15] It quoted, with approval, the conclusions in this regard of a Presidential Commission Report:[16]

The paucity of directly relevant cases makes characterization of the law in this area somewhat problematic, but certain points stand out. First, there is a presumption, strong but rebuttable, that parents are the appropriate decisionmakers for their infants. Traditional law concerning the family, buttressed by the emerging constitutional right of privacy, protects a substantial range of discretion for parents. Second, as persons unable to protect themselves, infants fall under the parens patriae power of the state. In the exercise of this authority, the state not only punishes parents whose conduct has amounted to abuse or neglect of their children but may also supervene parental decisions before they become operative to ensure that the choices made are not so detrimental to a child's interests as to amount to neglect and abuse.

. . . [A]s long as parents choose from professionally accepted treatment options the choice is rarely reviewed in court and even less frequently supervened. The courts have exercised their authority to appoint a guardian for a child when the parents are not capable of participating to the decisionmaking or when they have made decisions that evidence substantial lack of concern for the child's interests. Although societal involvement usually occurs under the auspices of governmental instrumentalities such as child welfare agencies and courts – the American legal system ordinarily relies upon the private initiative of individuals, rather than continuing governmental supervision, to bring the matter to the attention of legal authorities.[17]

What can be seen, then, is that the parental decision to consent or to withhold consent to medical treatment for their infants will be respected except in highly unusual and infrequently occurring circumstances.[18] The legal basis for this deferential attitude is grounded not only in the common law of the states, but also in the individual right of privacy which emanates from the Bill of Rights and is recognized as having a constitutional dimension. However, since such treatment decisions by parents necessarily arise in highly varied and individualized settings, the difficulty lies in gleaning a great deal of guidance, and in establishing any clear judicial precedent, for other similar, but inevitably different, treatment choice decisions.

The second and third of the recent cases to reach the US Supreme Court, involving the withholding of life-sustaining treatment from children, were ones in which the Court denied review.[19] Little can be read into this decision but, in both cases, the Court let stand the parents' decision not to consent to treatment of their handicapped child. In one case, commonly known as the 'Baby Doe' case, the infant in question had died by the time the case was presented to the Court and the issues raised were accordingly moot and presented no justiciable controversy.[20] Nonetheless, the Court could have granted review if it felt the decision, outlined below, to be clearly erroneous and/or that the issues were of significant dimension, calling for authoritative elucidation. The case arose in Indiana when the parents of a Downs syndrome infant refused consent to treatment proposed by the hospital physicians to correct an oesophageal obstruction which prevented oral feeding of the child. Apparently, other significant medical complications existed in the case, although they were not made public since the record in the case was ordered sealed.

In any event, on the day following the parents' non-consent to proposed medical treatment, the hospital sought court-imposed authority to treat over the wishes of the parents, through the appointment of a legal guardian for the child. Indiana, as is true in virtually all states,[21] had a parental neglect statute which was relied upon to seek removal of treatment authority from the parents. The trial court, following hearing, denied the hospital's request. It did, however, refer the matter to the child welfare authorities for investigation, and they, following review, declined to take issue with the ruling of the trial court. The Indiana Court of Appeals denied a request for immediate hearing, and on appeal to the Indiana Supreme Court, a petition for writ of mandamus was rejected.[22]

The fact that the US Supreme Court denied review in the now-famous 'Baby Doe' case is subject to differing interpretations. It may be suggested, however, that, in the absence of manifest abuse, the Court felt this to be an area of concern best left to individual decision-making between parents and physicians if at all possible; that adequate state laws on parental neglect are already in place to deal with cases of clear abuse or neglect; and that where the parents elect, in refusing consent to treatment, to follow the recommendations of one of two or more 'reasonable' medical judgements, their decision is legally acceptable.

Although not officially reported, it appears that Baby Doe suffered not just from Down's syndrome, but also from at least one other significant defect involving the heart which may not, in any event, have been amenable to surgical correction, or only at considerable risk. As a result, available medical opinion apparently differed as to the child's prognosis, even with correction of the oesophageal blockage. That being the case, it is likely that the Court concluded that it was inappropriate to overrule the parents where they had chosen between differing, but reasonable, medical judgements.

The other recent case where review was denied by the Supreme Court involved a 12-year old Downs Syndrome boy who also suffered from a congenital heart defect. Corrective surgery, involving only a 5–10 per cent risk of mortality was proposed to avoid a painful, degenerative process, resulting in premature death in some 20 years. The parents, who had institutionalized the boy, refused consent. The trial and appellate courts upheld their decision.[23] The Supreme Court acknowledged that, 'where parents fail to provide their children with adequate medical care, the state is justified to intervene',[24] so the decision not to intervene in this case seems somewhat incongruous. Although the decision was criticized, it was allowed to stand. No parental abuse or neglect was considered as proven.

Fortunately, two years later custody over the boy was awarded to concerned surrogate parents who authorised treatment of the heart defect, if still feasible. That decision was upheld on appeal.[25] The court was able to apply a broader standard of what was in the child's 'best interests' in the guardianship proceeding. This allowed a more favourable outcome for the child than did the earlier proceeding which, in effect, required overruling of the parents' non-treatment decision upon a finding of abuse or neglect. The decision reached in the subsequent guardianship proceeding is more in line with US legal precedent in this area. Thus, the Supreme Court's election to deny *certiorari* in the earlier proceeding is persuasive evidence of the deference it feels should be afforded parental decision-making and state adjudications in this area.

Constitutional underpinning for parental discretion

Much of the deference afforded the decisions of parents to refuse consent to medical treatment for their children stems from the US Constitution. No express right or provision exists, but a privacy right, implicit in the Bill of Rights, has been recognized as one which applies to 'matters relating to marriage, procreation, contraception, family relationships, and child rearing and education'.[26] It has been extended to include a woman's right to terminate her pregnancy,[27] and, apparently includes, generally, matters falling within 'the freedom to care for one's health and person'.[28] The idea is to promote and protect the 'integrity' of the family, of which child-rearing decisions are an important part.[29]

However, as with most constitutional rights afforded the individual, the rights and prerogatives of parents to decide upon treatment for their children are limited by several factors. Courts confronted with such cases apply a balancing test, giving weight to the often competing interests of the state and the child. The older the child, the greater influence his or her preference will have.[30] When the child is of an age to give an informed consent to treatment, it will normally be honoured notwithstanding parental wishes to the contrary. The issue is a factual one relating to the stage at which the child understands the nature and consequences of a treatment decision. No arbitrary age is deemed controlling. Obviously, the child's intelligence, understanding and the nature and complexity of the treatment decision will vary from case to case. However, normally if the child has attained age 14, it can be said that parental preferences will not be allowed to contradict the wishes of the child.[31]

The competing interest of greatest counterbalance to parental discretion is the state's interest in preserving healthy life. Where the life of the child can be saved, medical treatment will be ordered and the judgement of the state substituted for that of the parents. Parents are not given 'life and death authority over their children'.[32] The state, in its role of *parens patriae* has both the right and the duty to protect the health and physical well-being of its children. However, as noted, the justification for intervention must be substantial, the risk of harm to the child clear. Such is the case where, for example, blood or surgery is immediately necessary to save the life or preserve the health of the child, regardless of what philosophical or religious conviction may motivate the parents' non-consent. However, this principle, in practice, only applies in cases where return to, or maintenance of, healthy life is possible. Where the child is significantly handicapped, a double standard seems to apply and in these cases, parents are given much broader latitude. Subjective quality of life decisions, if supported by doctors – and even where not supported by some – [33] seem to be accepted.

Where parents fail to obtain medical treatment for an ill child because of their religious beliefs and the child dies, they may well be convicted of reckless homicide.[34] Why such action has apparently never occurred where parents decide to withhold treatment consent for a seriously disabled newborn is unclear, but it is suggestive of such a double standard.

Actions by the state courts

State courts have consistently overruled parental non-consent to medical treatment immediately necessary to save the life of their otherwise healthy child. The most noted cases are those where necessary blood transfusions are opposed by the parents on religious grounds. The courts have had little trouble in affirming that the state interest in preserving the child's life outweighs any parental privacy or religious freedom interests.[35] Whilst the Constitution guarantees parents full freedom in their religious *beliefs*, this does not extend to *actions* jeopardizing the life or health of others.[36] These are situations where the parents' actions are not supported by medical opinion.

Infants are unable to express their preferences for or against treatment. The standard then available is what is in the 'best interests' of the infant. This is to be an objective standard and is one based on what a 'reasonable' person would want in the circumstances – not necessarily what the infant would want, rather, what most *adult* people would want if they were in such a situation. It is a standard necessarily interpreted by adults, for infants. Albeit imperfect, the courts have long relied upon it as the best available means to decide what is best for the child. Not knowing his or her actual wishes, and an infant being unable to form such wishes knowingly, doing what most people in society consider right or reasonable is the only recourse of the law.[37]

Where the infant is in an irreversible coma, or in a persistent vegetative state such that no cognitive abilities are manifest and there is no reasonable chance for improvement, a parental decision to refuse consent to further treatment has been upheld.[38] In such cases the state's interest in preserving healthy life is of little weight, given the status and prognosis of the infant. The scales are tipped to uphold parental prerogatives here, given a competently established medical diagnosis and prognosis.

Where the infant has multiple and severe birth defects, such that he or she will be unable to survive regardless of treatment, the parents may refuse consent to further treatment, including medically induced provision of nourishment by intravenous feedings or surgical repair.[39] Such cases are often those involving severe neural tube defects or myelomeningocele. In one such case, however, hospital authorities were granted surgical authorization over the parents' refusal to allow treatment on showing that the child would, with surgical repair of her spinal lesion, have normal intellectual development, although physical defects causing incontinence and limitation of the lower extremities would remain. The court was persuaded that it was not a 'hopeless' case, the lesion was low on the spine and the child could expect to live a 'useful, fulfilling life'.[40]

The attitude of the attending physicians toward treatment has played a strong role in influencing court decisions. If the parental decision not to treat is supported by reasonable medical judgement, despite contrary opinion, it is unlikely the court will substitute its judgement for that of parents and physicians. Courts have not, for example, ordered treatment, in such instances, for infants suffering from Hodgkins disease,[41] myelomeningocele, microcephaly and hydrocephalus,[42] Down's syndrome accompanied by apparent serious coronary anomoly and intestinal blockage,[43] severe neural tube defect with exposed brain tissue mass,[44] and irreversible coma.[45]

Summary

What emerges from the fabric of the US cases, and limited statutory enactments, is that in the absence of clear benefit to the infant, supported by medical opinion, parental decisions to withhold treatment from severely handicapped infants will rarely be challenged and even more rarely overturned. Even where the infant's condition is life-threatening, the majority practice is that treatment will not be compelled if

1   the infant is irreversibly comatose;
2   treatment will only prolong inevitable death, expected to occur within the near future;
3   treatment will not permit the child to participate to any degree in human relationships or to interact with others because of severe mental retardation or dysfunction; or
4   treatment cannot accomplish survival of the infant without chronic, intolerable pain such as to make continued treatment inhumane.[46]

In a case that suggests the framework for category (4) above – albeit one concerning an elderly, nursing home patient – the New Jersey Supreme Court, best known for its landmark *Quinlan* judgement in 1976 – [47] recently held that life-sustaining treatment could properly be withdrawn from an elderly nursing home patient with multiple, serious illnesses where the patient's treatment desires were unknown if, (1) the burdens of continued treatment clearly outweighed its benefits, and (2) the 'recurring, unavoidable and severe pain of the patient's life with the treatment' made its continued imposition 'inhumane'.[48]

It can be said that only two quality of life considerations should ever justify non-treatment of a deformed infant: that is, where the treatment is futile or inhumane. Treatment is futile if it cannot reverse permanent unconsciousness (brain death or persistent vegetative state), forestall imminent death, or prevent pain so chronic and severe as to make treatment prolonging life inhumane. Value judgements enter here, since pain is subjective, but at some point, presumably, medicine can agree on such a condition, try as it might and justly should to avoid it.

In support of this strict position, several courts have held that, regardless of what the infant's prognosis might be, if medical treatment will salvage the infant's life and it is feasible or practical to undertake the treatment, it must be provided, regardless of the parents' wishes and the preferences of the attending physicians. As stated in one such case:

In the Court's opinion the issue before the Court is not the respective quality of the life to be preserved, but the medical feasibility of the proposed treatment compared with the almost certain risk of death should treatment be withheld. Being satisfied that corrective surgery is medically necessary and medically feasible, the Court finds that the defendants herein have no right to withhold such treatment and that to do so constitutes neglect in the legal sense.[49]

In another case, the infant, having suffered congenital rubella, was born with severe birth defects. Surgery was necessary to save the infant's life, even though it had a mortality risk of 50–60 per cent. In light of the risk of the surgery, the family refused consent. On petition by the attending physician, the court concluded that the infant's quality of life was not to be considered and that, ' . . . if there is any life-saving treatment available, it must be undertaken regardless of the quality of the life that will result'.[50]

Most US decisions allow the parents substantial latitude in electing to refuse consent to life-sustaining treatment for their severely handicapped infant. Where this once appeared to include Downs syndrome infants, this seems no longer to be the case. The same is true for infants suffering from spina bifida, but with low lesions which are treatable and will not impair relatively normal intellectual development. However, for those infants in irreversible coma, facing inevitable and imminent death, with severe neurological deficits preventing any cognitive interaction with those around them, or in those rare cases of unmanageable, intolerable pain, parents have refused and will refuse consent to treatment, physicians have supported and will support them, courts will rarely be petitioned and, if so, will not intervene. Nonetheless, in infrequent cases, courts will look only to the feasibility of the medical treatment proposed, not to the infant's level of existence with treatment. In those few cases, such a 'feasibility' approach by the judge will dictate that treatment go forward in all but the most hopeless and tragic cases.

British legal precedent

The overview

Whilst less precedent exists in Britain than in the USA, and whilst a different constitutional framework applies, the legal positions appear remarkably similar. The same general rule emerges, but not without qualification and even apparent contradiction. The rights of parents to control at infancy are recognized to yield over time to little more than advice as the child matures toward adulthood.[51] In England and Wales a child has the statutory right to consent (or, presumably, refuse consent) to medical treatment upon attaining age 16.[52] This, of course, is not to say that a child younger than 16 does not have the right or ability to consent, or refuse consent, to medical treatment if able to make an informed decision.[53] This is consistent with the law on the subject in Canada,[54] the USA[55] and Scotland.[56]

Considerable legal deference is accorded physicians' treatment decisions involving infants. The courts are the ultimate arbiters of what is and what is not an acceptable medical practice standard. Whilst ' . . . the law will not permit the medical profession to play God',[57] there is still great reluctance to gainsay a physician's decision not actively to treat a birth-defective infant.

In the UK, as in the USA, the intentional taking of life, no matter how altruistic the motive, is criminal homicide.[58] Furthermore, the fact of limited expected life span, or the likelihood of imminent death from pre-existing natural causes, provides neither excuse nor justification for homicide.[59] Finally, neither the consent, nor the earnest plea, of the victim provides insulation from criminality.[60] Of course, the latter plea is not relevant in the instance of a newborn incapable of such an expression of intent.

Clearly relevant, however, is the issue of whether omissions, the failure to undertake treatment necessary to sustain the infant, would be treated any differently from an affirmative act causing death. Until the physician takes on a case, he or she has no duty to treat. However, once the physician–patient relationship commences, a legal duty arises. Where a legal duty to treat or care for one in need exists, then the law will impose criminal liability for a failure to act to fulfil the duty.[61] Child neglect or abuse statutes are a good example of this.[62]

With a handicapped newborn, then, the critical question is whether there exists an affirmative legal duty to treat in the face of severe disability and parental objection. Where the physician believes, in good faith, that treatment is not indicated, and where that belief is supported by a responsible body of medical opinion, it is very unlikely that criminal liability will emanate from the decision not to treat.[63]

The Arthur case

In the UK, there has been reported only one recent prosecution of a physician for withholding medical treatment from a seriously handicapped infant. The case demonstrated the great reluctance of the English criminal system to convict a physician for electing not to treat, where that decision is supported by other responsible physicians as acceptable medical practice and is consistent with the wishes of the parents. The decision not to treat was made because the child was born handicapped with Down's syndrome. Apparently, defects of the brain, heart and lung also complicated the infant's prognosis, although it does not appear that death was imminent if active or aggressive surgical repair and treatment had been undertaken.

In this case, *Regina* v. *Arthur*,[64] the physician ordered 'nursing care only' for the Downs infant. The parents had been consulted and did not wish the infant to survive. Water, but no food was given, and the infant died some 69 hours later. The jury refused to convict of murder, having been instructed, 'I imagine that you will think long and hard before concluding that eminent doctors have evolved standards that amount to committing a crime'.[65] That charge was not far from a directed verdict. Evidence in the case showed parental non-consent, as well as expert testimony that Dr Arthur's conduct fell within generally accepted medical practice. The jury acquitted him of the charge (which was reduced to attempted murder in the course of the trial).

It seems clear that the intent was for the infant to die. The medical chart entry read, 'Parents do not wish it to survive'. But, as opined by Lord Scarman in the 'Gillick'[66] case, 'The bona fide exercise by a doctor of his clinical judgement must be a complete negation of the guilty mind [*mens rea*] which is an essential ingredient of the criminal offence. . . .'[67] What we have in the Arthur case is, in effect, as has been said,[68] application of the 'Bolam'[69] principle of civil non-liability to a criminal proceeding if a doctor acts in accordance with a responsible body of medical opinion and practice.

R. v. *Arthur* appears to have presented facts and issues remarkably similar to those raised in the Baby Doe case in the USA.[70] The contexts were different, one criminal, one civil, but the outcome the same. The infant's condition was remarkably similar in each. Whilst over-generalization is unwise, the cases suggest that it matters not a great deal on which side of the Atlantic you are, if you are asking courts to compel treatment or juries to convict in such cases. Both are most unlikely where:

1   parents refuse consent to treatment;
2   the attending physician concurs;
3   a responsible body of medical opinion is in agreement with the decision;
4   the infant suffers birth-defects involving the central nervous system which imply mental retardation or dysfunction; and

5   some other significant birth defect is present which is not readily
    amenable to surgical correction.

Re B (A Minor)

However, where Down's syndrome alone is presented, treatment
will and should be undertaken.[71] An English court so ordered when
presented prospectively with the request to authorize surgery to
remove an intestinal blockage (readily amenable to surgery) in a
Downs syndrome infant *Re B*.[72] The decision seems correct. It puts
the law where it should be. Mere mental retardation, of uncertain
degree, cannot be the basis for withholding feasible, life-saving
medical treatment.

Conclusions

It is difficult to reconcile *Arthur* and *Re B*. The degree of complication
in the condition of the infant in *Arthur* was, apparently, greater
and less amenable to surgical correction than that of the infant in
Re B, although it is not clear that Dr Arthur was aware of the extent
of the child's handicaps at the time the decision not to treat was
made. However, the more telling differences may simply be the
context in which each case arose. In one, prospective action was
taken to save a clearly salvageable infant. In the other, a noted
physician was charged with murder for following the wishes of the
parents and acting in accordance with accepted medical ethics as
voiced by at least a responsible part of the medical community. A
jury is simply not disposed to second-guess the parents after the
fact in such circumstances and to impose the severe sanction of
homicide guilt and conviction upon a respected physician.

The reported decision of the Director of Public Prosecutions not
to prosecute in some extreme cases,[73] and the noticeable lack of
prosecution in other such cases, despite the known incidence of
such birth defects,[74] suggest a strong reluctance to challenge medical
practice in this area in Britain, as in America. Unlike Downs
syndrome, the birth defect of spina bifida carries with it the likelihood of significant pain and early mortality in more than half of
the cases.

What seems to emerge is that Downs syndrome infants, who can
survive without chronic pain and can relate to their environment
and others around them, will be ordered treated if refusals to do
so come to the attention of the authorities. However, where more
severe neural tube defects present the prospect of chronic and
severe pain, or the inability, due to severe mental dysfunction, to
relate to other people, then non-treatment decisions of parents

and physicians will rarely be challenged and even more rarely overturned or prosecuted.

This is not to say, however, that parents will be permitted to take decisions which are clearly not in the best interests of their children, nor that birth defects will necessarily provide easy justification for broader parental discretion over treatment decisions. For example, in Re D.[75], an 11 year-old girl's parent sought authorization for her to be sterilized because of mental retardation, epilepsy and emotional instability. However, the girl was felt capable of marriage. The mother asserted that the girl would be incapable of caring for a child, who might also inherit the defects in question. In rejecting the request, the English court pointed out that compelling sterilization would deprive the girl of her basic human right to procreate, the procedure was not therapeutically necessary, and was not in her 'best interests'. Saying the treatment was not in the child's 'best interests' was conclusionary rather than an aid to analysis. Presumably, the court felt that the heavy burden of demonstrating harm to the young girl or an eventual offspring could not be met in sufficient degree as to warrant interference with her right to procreational freedom. Other, less radical, forms of contraception may have been felt feasible. The court also pointed out that treatment which is not solely therapeutic does not rest solely within the doctor's clinical judgement.[76]

The case reaches an outcome consistent with its US counterparts, recognizing that the authority of parents over medical treatment for their children will be carefully scrutinized by the courts to ensure that what is deemed to be in the child's best interests is accomplished. It is one thing to do this with a healthy child, but quite another for normal adults, in the person of doctors, parents and ultimately judges, to decide whether it is best for severely handicapped infants to be treated or whether the severity of their handicap somehow makes non-treatment in their best interests. This seems a nearly impossible task except for a narrow area of application. In the absence of intolerable pain or pemanent unconsciousness, how can it be said an infant would rather be dead? How can anyone presume to know?

In the UK, contrary to the prevailing position in the USA, infants are given the right to sue for a reduction in the quality of their life, if negligence and causation are proved. This apparently is a common law right in Scotland and the result of statute in England.[77] If such a right exists, then it can be argued that it is not proper to terminate infant life on the basis that defects are such as to create an unacceptable quality of life for the child.[78] If the infant can sue for diminished quality of life, then the right to live that life, however impaired, seems to be at least implicitly recognized. Thus, others have no right to prevent enjoyment of that impaired life either by action or inaction.

This conclusion seems proper, parental decision-making rights to the contrary notwithstanding, *provided* the infant has some potential for independent existence. However, if the infant is irreversibly comatose, saddled with chronic pain of intolerable or inhumane degree not amenable to control, or possesses – because of severe neurological deficit – no cognitive ability to relate to and react with others around him or her, then it may be concluded that parental choices in respect of treatment for their own infants, when consistent with the professional judgement of the attending physicians, acting in good faith, could outweigh the interests of infants to continued medical maintenance at such a low level of existence. Nonetheless this last conclusion might well be thought to demand that the decisions of parents or physicians should be subject to review, especially since they do not cease to be subjective simply because they are readily intelligible. In effect, what is argued for here is humane decision-making, rather than exclusively for parental or medical rights as such.

Conflicting interests of parents, physicians and infant

Parents

Parents share in the conception of the child. The mother carries the child *in utero* and undergoes profound physical and emotional changes as a consequence. Often the decision to bear the child is planned and truly elective. On other occasions, perhaps due to ignorance, poverty or religious practice, it is not.

In either case, the parents have the moral, physical and societal responsibility to care for and raise the child. It is they who will most immediately feel, see, and experience each and every day, the deficiencies or defects of their handicapped newborn. So too their emotional and financial resources may be taxed, perhaps to the detriment or deprivation of other family members and loved ones. Some will cope without complaint. Some will be enriched, perhaps beyond the birth of a healthy child. Some, however, will not, or will fear that they cannot cope or that they should not have to cope. The abilities of each parent will be different in relating to and nurturing such a child. Should not these parents, to whom we trust all our children – the future of our society – be entitled to decide if the degree of defect exhibited by their newborn is too severe a burden for them to shoulder? Are they not the most interested, the most involved, the most affected by the decision?

Apparently, a woman cannot be prohibited from aborting her foetus, whether viable or not, if necessary to preserve her health.[79] If so, then can she (as well as the father) make a case not actively to treat a severely deformed newborn whose needs and constant condition will, they genuinely believe, be harmful to their ongoing health? Is it more harmful to society to force such newborns upon shunning parents and to burden further a medical system of limited resources, than to permit parents to elect against treatment, with the advice and concurrence of the attending physicians?

Abortion, at least in part, is permitted to avoid saddling parents with unwanted offspring. Is this not a component of personal, marital and familial autonomy, a value that should be extended to certain limited and atypical instances of severely deformed newborns? Obviously limits must be imposed, but should they not seek to maximize the freedom of choice of parents, and physicians?

Physicians

Physicians' freedoms, ethics and professional judgement may, however, conflict with the rights or interests of parents. When the parents feel they cannot cope, and do not want the child, the doctor may yet feel that he or she can, and should actively, treat the child. Yet, without parental consent, he or she cannot – except in emergency situations which, arguably, many of these cases may be. Recourse may then be necessary to courts. The courts have recognized that protecting the physician's proper exercise of his or her professional judgement is an important objective of both the law and society.[80] The physician's first and strongest medical mandate is to heal, to cure, and to repair. This will often translate itself into a strong desire actively and aggressively to treat a defective newborn, even in the face of parental objection and the need to resort to the courts. If the doctor feels he or she can relieve pain, improve the prognosis, why should parents be able to interfere with his or her desire and duty to help the child? Is not his or her ethic to save life sullied if it cannot be done in cases where it is feasible, but unwanted by the parents? The physician may understand the infant's potential for meaningful survival better than the parents whose shame, grief or depression may seriously impair their ability to make an informed decision.

Of course, it must not be forgotten that not all can be cured. All die. The physician has the compelling mandate to comfort as well as cure. If pain can be alleviated, comfort given, but life is inadvertently shortened, there seems no wrong.[81]

The infant

But what of the interests of the infant? Who speaks for the infant? Does not each child have the right to live, regardless of handicap? Who can presume to say that non-existence is better than impaired existence? Whilst the state is there to protect the infant, most of the decisions which have been discussed occur well away from the eye of the state. Only when a disgruntled member of the medical staff takes issue are they aired publicly. Yet compelling treatment is not a simple solution. We do it without knowing if it is wanted or may be later regretted by the infant. If treatment enables survival, what pain will come with it? What will be the state's involvement in providing for that child if the parents will not? And if the states' finite financial and personnel resources are committed to the growing infant, as seems proper, what other lives and societal interest suffer loss?

In conclusion

Much about life and death may seem unfair and haphazard. Loved ones are taken prematurely without reason or explanation. Some are blessed with healthy children, others are not. Whilst not fully comprehending life and death, we must not lose reverence for all human life, handicapped or not. All should have equal opportunity to survive. However, if we are not arbitrary and not discriminatory, is it not reasonable and proper to conclude that some lives may be allowed to come and pass without active medical intervention if they possess too little of what we understand to set us apart and give life meaning?

If newborns are irreversibly comatose, will never have cognition of life and those around them, or if they are conscious, but so devoid of intellect and cognition that they cannot relate to other people or to their environment, as determined by competent medical diagnosis, then parents should not be forced aggressively to treat them in order to sustain them. The same is true if death in the very near future cannot be avoided and treatment is a futile gesture that cannot measurably expand a conscious existence of tolerable pain.

It seems proper that the decision to treat aggressively, or to offer only comfort care, in the case of a severely handicapped infant coming within the general parameters mentioned, must be made promptly after birth. However, this is, at best, a difficult time. It will probably be the time when the parents are most affected by their emotional reaction to the infant's birth, by shock, fear, disappointment, guilt, uncertainty or shame. Also, in many cases prognosis will not be certain.

Nonetheless, the physician must disclose all material facts concerning the infant's diagnosis, prognosis with and without treatment, the risks and side-effects of treatment, alternatives of care available and, inevitably, the physician's appraisal of the degree of pain and suffering the child will endure both with and without treatment, as well as the degree to which the child will be able to relate cognitively to his or her environment and to those around him or her. A second, consulting, opinion from a qualified neonatologist or paediatrician should be solicited, obtained, explained to the parents and entered in the medical record.

One prominent physician, experienced in such cases, has suggested that only nursing or comfort care, excluding antiobiotics or intravenous feeding, should be given to infants exhibiting certain recognized symptoms of severe neurological deficit, but that if the infant survives beyond six months it should then be actively treated because of its unexpected potential for long-term survival.[82] Just as the rights of the foetus increase during pregnancy,[83] so too it would seem do the rights of the infant to an independent existence – regardless of severity of birth defects – the longer the infant survives.

When the infant exhibits the ability to survive, without intolerable pain, in a conscious state, with the cognitive potential for some interpersonal relationships, and death is not irreversible and imminent, then the right of parents and physicians to elect against life-sustaining treatment should not be available or legally countenanced. Whilst 'imminent' is a slippery, ill-defined term, death within one year or less, regardless of treatment, seems a workable criterion.[84]

It may be that statutory limits are advisable in this area. Certainly, albeit at the risk of interfering with medical judgement, they could provide some certainty, by placing strict time limits on postparatum decisions not to treat.[85] However, accepted guidelines for medical treatment in such cases would be more flexible and preferable.[86]

In cases where the informed, joint decision of parents and physicians is not actively to treat, comfort care must always be given. This should include warmth, sanitation, hydration and nutrition if capable of being taken by mouth, and medication for pain. It is possible that the latter may hasten death, but its administration is permissible if intended to control pain. As the jury was instructed by Mr Justice Devlin in the 1957 murder prosecution of one Dr Adams:

If the first purpose of medicine, the restoration of health, can no longer be achieved there is still much for a doctor to do, and he is entitled to do all that is proper and necessary to relieve pain and suffering, even if the measures he takes may incidentally shorten life. But it remains the fact, and it remains the law, that no doctor, nor any man, no more in the case of the dying than of the healthy, has the right deliberately to cut the thread of life.[87]

Most legal precedent has refused to accept the proposition that claims may be made for being allowed to be born with deformities, rather than not to be born at all. However, some precedent has suggested it cannot be absolutely said that life, no matter how impaired, is always preferable to nonexistence.[88] Numerous US jurisdictions, by statute or case law, have recognized the right of a competent adult to choose to die by declining life-sustaining treatment when they are terminally and incurably ill and can no longer tolerate the invasiveness of the medical care necessary to sustain them.[89] The same is true when the patient is incompetent to decide, but has expressed him or herself clearly on the subject prior to the onset of a last debilitating illness or coma-induced incompetence.[90] Even where no expression of desire has been competently expressed, where the burdens of treatment clearly outweigh its benefit and where its continued imposition would be inhumane due to severe and chronic pain, it is not legally required to preserve an existence without regard to its severe impairment.[91]

These decisions recognize that individuals may choose, or be presumed to have chosen, death over continued, but severely impaired, existence. Rights of self-determination, personal autonomy and privacy underpin this freedom to choose. Yet it is one thing to allow death to occur where life has been lived and where adult values may be applied in deciding or upholding what another wants done, or what is reasonably believed to be in his or her 'best interests' under the unfortunate circumstances of an unremitting terminal illness or unconsciousness; it is quite another to apply these principles to a newborn infant.

By recognizing the aforesaid rights of adults – competent or incompetent – to die without undue or inhumane prolongation of death, society is recognizing that its interest in preserving life yields, at some point, to the right of personal freedom and dignity. It does so when the life to be preserved is of little value because of its short remaining duration, possible only with great pain or dehumanizing medical intervention, or lack of interrelational or interpersonal cognition (chronic vegetative state or severe brain dysfunction).

If such decisions are accepted in the case of adults, should not infants have similar rights? It would seem acceptable to withhold treatment in such limited instances from infants, provided:

1 the diagnosis and prognosis are competently made;
2 a corroborative and qualified second medical opinion has been obtained;
3 the parents, after full disclosure and deliberation have elected to withhold consent to further treatment;
4 there is no issue of bad faith or ill motive (that is, to cover up professional malpractice); and
5 the attending physicians, in the exercise of their professional medical judgement and ethics, concur with the parental decision.

Whilst the 'best interests' standard may properly be applied to adults, and perhaps to older children, it really has no application to newborns. It is premised on what most reasonable people would want done under the circumstances. Such substitute judgements can be made for people who have attained an age where others – the legendary 'reasonable men' of tort and delict law – have experienced that maturity and can conclude from their own experience what most would want at that age. However, no one recalls what they wanted or thought best for themselves at birth.

So, in deciding for infants on the basis of their best interests, we are deciding simply what *we* think is best for them. This is not necessarily what *is* best for them, nor what they would think best for themselves if able to form and express an informed choice. We cannot know the answer to these inquiries. It would be more honest to couch newborn non-treatment choices of parents not in the context of the infant's 'best interests', but rather based on the level of physiological existence which treatment will enable the infant to sustain. What the courts (and in some select few cases the juries) have said, in effect, is that where the infant's physiological level of existence falls below a certain standard, we will not second-guess parents' decisions not to treat, where concurred with by the attending physicians.

That standard, that minimum level of physiological existence below which parents' and physicians' non-treatment choices will not be disturbed, exists where the infant:

1 faces inevitable death in the near future, which will only be prolonged by painful or invasive medical treatment which cannot cure or offer benefits (improvement in physical living conditions) which outweight its burdens;
2 is irreversibly comatose or, because of severe neurological deficit

(anencephaly, encephaloceles or myelomeningocele), is incapable of sufficient cognition to relate to others around him or her and to his or her environment; or

3 is the victim of such chronic and severe pain so as to make the imposition of treatment inhumane.

In such situations, the value we assign as a society to the rights of parents and the judgements of physicians outweighs the value we assign to such miserable levels of physiological existence for the infant. Since these values conflict, we must assign them weight before we can determine which prevails. Few would argue that in these very limited, but wrenching and intensely personal, situations, the balance has in general been properly struck on the parents' side of the scale, where the decision made can be seen to be humane. As was noted earlier, although an apparent vindication of parental or medical rights, it is the light of humanity which crucially determines the status of the decision, even where the choice made results in the death of an infant.

Of course, in those cases where there is disagreement among the treating physicians between physicians and parents, or between parents, as to the proper treatment decision for the infant, treatment should continue unless and until the judicial appointment of a guardian or conservator with express authority to withhold consent to further treatment. Courts faced with differences of opinion in such cases are unlikely to authorize withdrawal of withholding of treatment except in the clearest instances of hopelessness.

We must tread softly and thoughtfully in this thicket. Abuse must be avoided. Error should be on the side of treatment. However, we must recognize the limitations on the abilities of parents and physicians to care for those few lives that are simply not salvageable to a condition which allows for the capacity to relate to others and to their environment – those most fundamental indicia of human life.

The law should be flexible enough to permit humane decision-making in these cases, but certain enough to prevent abuse. The evolving common law seems to have allowed this. Inevitably, however, judge–made law, in such an emotional and individualized context, will result in inconsistency and uncertainty at times. This may be the price to be paid for the flexibility that is needed. Given the few cases of reported abuse or harm, the current system, with all its imperfections, may be satisfactory, though its fairness, consistency and acceptability would be enhanced by clearer articulation of non-treatment standards and guidelines by the medical profession in such cases.[92]

Setting precise standards is probably not possible. At what point, for example, does an impaired infant's cognitive potential become so low that he or she will not be able to love or be loved,[93] to realized the potential for human relationships,[94] or to interact with his or her environment or with other people?[95] These are guidelines which must, of necessity, allow for some latitude in their application. However, this is not undesirable, for those who apply them – parents and physicians – are best suited to do so. No one can be presumed to want more what is best for the child than the parents. No one can be presumed better able to evaluate condition and prognosis than the attending physicians. Together they have, with rare exception, applied these standards well, without evident abuse. One is an effective and moderating balance for the other. In those rare instances of abuse, existing child abuse and neglect reporting laws,[96] and the local infrastructure to enforce them, should be adequate protection for the child. Society and its legal system can ask for no more.

Notes

1   *Fed. reg.* V 50. No. 72 (4/15/85), p. 14886
2   Freeman. 'The short-sided treatment of myelomeningocele: long-term case report', **53** *Pediatrics*, 1974, 31 1.
3   Duff and Campbell, 'Moral and ethical dilemmas in the special-care nursery, **289** *New England Journal of Medicine* 1973, 890.
4   C.f. Duff and Campbell, loc. cit., note 3 *supra.*
5   C.f. Freeman, loc cit., note 2, *supra.*
6   *Meyer* v. *Nebraska* (1928) 262 US 390, 399.
7   *Bonner* v. *Moran* (D C Cir., 1941) 126 Fed 2d 121, 122
8   *Becker* v. *Schwartz* (1978, NY) 386 NE 2d 807, 812
9   Cf. Smith, 'Disabled newborns and the federal child abuse amendments: tenuous protection', **37**, *Hastings Law Journal* 1986, 765, 780
10 See Arras, 'Toward an ethic of ambiguity', *Hastings Center Report* 1984 25. Smith, loc. cit. note 9, *supra.*
11 S. 504 Rehabilitation Act 1973, 87 Stat 394, 29 USC (United States Code), s 794.
12 45 CFR (Code of Federal Regulations) s. 84, 55 (1985).
13 US v. *University Hospital*, (1984, 2d Cir) 729 F 2d 144.
14 *Bowen* v. *American Hospital Association* (1986) US, 106 S. Ct. 2101.
15 106 S. Ct. 2113.
16 Ibid., quoting the *Report of the President's Commission for the Study of Ethical Problems in Medicare & Biomedical & Behavioral Resarch*, US Govt. Printing Office, 1983.
17 Ibid., pp. 212–14.
18 A conclusion recognized by the government in the Bowen case, note 15 *supra,* 2113.
19 *Infant Doe* v. *Bloomington Hospital* (1983) 464 US 961, 104 S. Ct. 394; *Re B.* (1979) 445 US 949, 100 S. Ct. 1597.
20 *Infant Doe* v *Bloomington Hospital, supra cit.* note 19.
21 California Penal Code s. 270, for example, makes criminal the acts of a parent if he or she 'willfully omits, without lawful excuse, to furnish *necessary*

clothing, food, shelter or *medical attendance*, or other remedial care for his or her child'.

22 *In re Infant Doe*, no. GU 8204–009A (Monroe County Cir. Ct., 4/12/82). (Court of Appeals): *State ex. rel. Infant Doe v. Baker*, no. 4825140 (5/12/82), (Indiana Supreme Court).

23 *Re Phillip B.* (1979) 92 Cal App 3d 796.

24 Ibid., 92 Cal App 3d 801.

25 *Guardianship of Phillip B.* (1983) 139 Cal App 3d 407.

26 *Paul v Davis* (1976) 424 US 693, 96 S. Ct. 1155 (rehrg. den.).

27 *Roe v Wade* (1973) 410 US 113, 93 S. Ct. 1409.

28 *Doe v. Bolton* (1973) 410 US 179, 93 S. Ct. 739 (rehrg. den.), (Mr Justice Douglas concurring).

29 *L. v Matheson* (1981) 450 US 398, 101 S. Ct. 1164.

30 *Re Phillip B, supra cit*, note 23.

31 For example, the California guardianship statute requires the consent of a minor of 14 years or older to medical treatment decisions, unless overriden by court order or emergency need to save life or limb (California Probate Code s. 2353). Medical treatment decisions include decisions not to consent to treatment; see *Dority v. Superior Court* (1983) 145 Cal App 3d 273.

32 *Custody of Minor* (1978, Mass) 379 NE 2d 1053, 1063; for further discussion, see Sher, E. J., 'Choosing for children; adjuciating medical care disputes between parents and the state', **58** *New York University Law Review'*, 1983, 157.

33 Cf. notes 18 and 22, *supra*.

34 *Hall v State* (1986, Ind.) 493 NE 2d 433.

35 *State v. Perricone* (1962, NJ) 181 A 2d 751, cert den. 371 US 890, 83 S. Ct. 189.

36 *Application of President and Directors of Georgetown College Int.* (1964, DC) 331 F 2d 1000, cert den 377 US 978, 74 S. Ct. 1883.

37 For discussion of the concept of the 'best interests' of the child see, Goldstein, J., Freud, A., and Solnit, A. J., *Beyond the Best Interests of the Child*, London, Collier Macmillan, 1973

38 *Guardianship of Barry* (1985, Fla App) 455 So 2d 365; *Re L. H. R.* (1984, GA) 321 SE 2d 716; *Re W.* (1982, La) 424 So 2d 1015).

39 *Matter of Baby F* (1983, Coos Co. Ore, Cir Ct) No J 928 (occipital encephalocele); see also notes 13 and 22 *supra*.

40 *Re Cicero* (1979, NY) 421 NYS 2d 965, 967.

41 *Re Hofbauer* (1979, NY) 393 NE 2d 1009.

42 *Weber v. Stony Brook Hospital* (1983, NY) 456 NE 2d 1186, cert den 464 US 1027, 104 S. Ct. 560; *U.S. v University Hospital*, note 13, *supra*.

43 *In Re Infant Doe; State ex rel. Infant Doe v Baker, supra cit*, note 22.

44 *Matter of Baby F. supra cit*, note 39.

45 *Guardianship of Barry; Re W., supra cit*, note 38.

46 Mason, J. K. and Meyers, D. W., 'Parental choice and selective non-treatment of deformed new-borns: a view from mid-atlantic', **12** *Journal of Medical Ethics*, 67 1986; Federal Child Abuse Prevention and Treatment Act of 1974, as amended, 45 CFR s.1340. 15(b)(2), (1984). In *U.S.* v. *University Hospital, supra cit.*, note 13, the appeals court affirmed non-treatment, observing that the infant's cerebral disabilities raised 'an extremely high risk that the child would be so severely retarded that she would never interact with her environment or with other people', (decision approved, *Bowen* v. *American Hospital Association, supra cit.*, note 14.

47 *In Re Quinlan*, 429 US 922 (1976).

48 *Re Conroy* (1985, NJ) 486 A 2d 1209, 1232.

49 *Maine Medical Center v. Houle* (1974) Cumberland County (Me.) Superior Court No. 74–145.

50 *In Re McNulty* (1978) Essex County (Mass.) Probate Court no. 1960.
51 *Hewer* v. *Bryant* [1969] 3 All ER 578, 582 (Denning, MR).
52 Family Law Reform Act 1969, s. 8(1).
53 *Gillick* v. *West Norfolk & Wisbech Area Health Authority* [1985] 3 All ER 402; [1985] 3 All ER 830; see Williams, G., 'The Gillick saga', **135** *New Law Journal*, 1985, 1156, 1179.
54 *Johnston v. Wellesley Hospital* (1970) 17 DLR (3d) 139.
55 *Baird* v. *Atty. Gen.* (1977, Mass) 360 NE 2d 288; *Younts* v. *St. Francis Hospital* (1970, Kan) 469 P 2d 330.
56 Norrie, K. McK., 'The Gillick case and parental rights in Scots law', *Scots Law Times* 1985 p. 157; *Murray* v. *Fraser* 1916 SC. 623.
57 *The Lancet*, 14 November 1981, pp. 1101–2; Mason and Meyers, *loc. cit.*, note 46 *supra*.
58 Hume, *Commentaries*, vol. 1, ch.1, p. 25; Smith, T. B., 'Law, professional ethics and the human body', *Scots Law Times* (News) 1950 pp. 245, 246; *Rex* v. *Simpson* (1965) 41 Cr. App. R. 218, 84 LJKB 1893.
59 See discussion of the prosecution for murder in 1957 of Dr John Bodkin Adams in Williams, G., *The Sanctity of Life and the Criminal Law*, London, Faber & Faber Ltd., 1958, pp. 288–9.
60 *H. M. Advocate* v. *Rutherford*, 1947 JC 1; Meyers, D., *The Human Body & The Law*, Edinburgh, The University Press, 1970, p. 146.
61 *Regina* v. *Instan* (1893) 1 QB 450; *Regina* v. *Arthur* (1981), discussed by Mason and Meyers, *loc cit.*, note 46 *supra*.
62 The Children Act 1975, s. 85; Children and Young Persons Act 1969, s. 1; Children and Young Persons Act 1933, s. 1; Children and Young Persons (Scotland) Act 1937, s. 12; Social Work (Scotland) Act 1968, ss. 32–44.
63 Skegg, P., *Law, Ethics and Medicine*, Oxford, Clarendon Press, 1984, p. 146; McLean, S. A. M. and Maher, G., *Medicine, Morals and the Law*, Aldershot, Gower, 1983 (reprinted 1985), p. 71.
64 Reported in *The Times*, 6 November 1981.
65 See Brahams, D. and Brahams, M., 'R. v. Arthur – is legislation appropriate?', *78 Law Society, Gazette*, 1981, p. 1342.
66 See note 53, *supra*.
67 *Gillick, supra cit.*, note 53 *supra*.
68 Mason and Meyers, *loc cit* note 46, *supra*: see also McLean and Maher, *op. cit.*, note 63 *supra* ch. 4.
69 *Bolam* v. *Friern Hospital Mgt. Committee* [1957] 1 All ER 118.
70 *supra cit.*
71 *The Lancet* (editorial), 1981, p. 1085; Report of the *President's Commission*, note 16 *supra* at p. 219.
72 *In Re B (a minor)* [1981] 1 WLR 1421; *The Lancet*, (1981), pp. 413, 1102.
73 *The Times*, 6 October 1981; discussed in Mason, J. K. and McCall Smith, R. A., *Law and Medical Ethics*, 2nd edn, London, Butterworths, 1987.
74 Myelomeningocele, for example occurs in about 1 in 1,000 live births. In severe cases, decisions are reached by physicians and parents not to treat. This has been a known and admitted practice for many years; Lorber, 'Selective treatment of myelomeningocele; to treat or not to treat', *53 Pediatrics* 1974, 307; Lorber; 'Results of treatment of myelomeningocele' 13 *Developmental Medicine and Child Neurology*, 1971 279; Duff and Campbell, note 3, *supra*.
75 *Re D.*, (1976) *Fam* 186 (English Law Reports, Family Division).
76 But see later decisions such as *Re Be* (Sterilisation [1987] 2 All ER 206 (C.A.); also *The Times*, 17 March 1987 (H.L.); and T.v.T. and Anon, *The Times*, 11 July 1987.
77 Scottish Law Commission, *Liability for Ante-Natal Injury*, Cmnd. 5371, 1973,

applying the equitable principles of the Roman Law; Congenital Disabilities (Civil Liability) Act 1976 (England–Wales).

78 McLean and Maher, note, note 63 *supra*, p. 69.
79 *Roe* v. *Wade. supra cit.*, note 27 (the state may regulate and even proscribe abortion during the third trimester of pregnancy, unless it is necessary to preserve the life or health of the mother).
80 *Thornburgh* v. *American College of Obstetricians and Gynecologists* (1986) US, 106 S. Ct. 2169, 2180
81 see note 59, *supra*.
82 See McCormick, 'To save or let die – the dilemma of modern medicine', **229** *JAMA*, 1974, 172.
83 *Roe* v. *Wade, supra cit.*, note 27.
84 Mason and Meyers, note 46 *supra*.
85 *Lorber, loc. cit.*, note 74, *supra* see also, Freeman, *loc. cit.* note 2 *supra*.
86 See proposals made by Mason, J. K. and McCall Smith, R. A., *Law and Medical Ethics*, 2nd edn, London, Butterworths, 1987, at p. 115.
87 Cf. Mason and Meyers, *loc. cit*, note 46, *supra*.
88 See Williams, *op cit.*, note 59, *supra*.
89 *Continental Cas. Co.* v. *Empire Cas. Co.* (1985, Colo App) 713 Pac 2d 384; *Turpin* v. *Sortini* (1982) 31 Cal. 3d 220.
90 See, for example, *Bouvia* v. *Superior Court* (1986) 179 Cal App 3d 1127; *Matter of Farrell* (1986, NJ Chancery) 514 Atl 2d 1342; see generally, Meyers, D. W., *Medico-Legal Implications of Death and Dying* Rochester, NY, Lawyers Cooperative Publishing Co., 1981, chs. 10 and 12.
91 *Barber* v. *Superior Court* (1983) 147 Cal App 3d 1006; *John F. Kennedy Memorial Hospital* v. *Bludworth* (1984, Fla) 452 So 2d 921.
92 For further discussion, see Mason and Meyers, *loc. cit*, note 46, *supra*.
93 Cf. Freeman, *loc. cit.*, note 2 *supra*.
94 Cf. McCormick, *loc cit.*, note 82 *supra*.
95 Cf. *U.S.* v. *University Hospital, supra cit.*, note 13; Mason and Meyers, *loc. cit.*, note 46 *supra*.
96 see notes 21 and 62 *supra*.

6 Sterilizing people with mental handicaps

CHRISTOPHER HEGINBOTHAM

On 30 April 1987 the House of Lords unanimously dismissed an appeal against an Appeal Court ruling to allow the sterilization of a young mentally handicapped woman just before her eighteenth birthday.[1] The celebrated case of 'Jeanette' (now formally reported as *Re B*) has done more than any in recent years to raise concern about the treatment of those unable, for whatever reason, to give informed consent to invasive or non-therapeutic procedures. This chapter will discuss the ethical issues involved in sterilization, consider the legal difficulties – especially in relation to non-competent adults – and suggest some criteria which might apply generally.

Jeanette was born in 1969, the second of five children. The father subsequently left home and took no further part in the ensuing proceedings. In 1973 the local authority took out a care order and the child lived for much of her time in local authority homes. She is of low intellectual ability and is described as having the intellectual level of a child of two or three, but able to perform domestic skills appropriate to a child of five or six. She can dress herself, attend to her menstruation, but appears not to understand traffic or money and is therefore allowed out very little. She suffers from epilepsy which is controlled by drugs, is moody and can be aggressive or violent. Psychotropic medication is sometimes given. In particular she has a high pain threshold and would, it is thought, unpick any surgical wound. She is overweight, has high blood pressure, and certain oral or injectible contraceptives are contra-indicated.[2]

Sunderland Borough Council, supported by Jeanette's mother, applied to the High Court for wardship so that sterilization could take place. Jeannette had been showing signs of 'sexual awakening' – a term not defined publicly but probably referring to masturbation

– and which should not be taken to imply a likelihood of sexual relations. Nonetheless her carers felt that reasonable freedom from supervision entailed a risk of pregnancy, which could only be avoided by contraception. The options were presented as:

(a) oral progesterone taken daily for the rest of her reproductive life, or
(b) sterilization by occlusion of the fallopian tubes, which would almost certainly be irreversible.

Injectible contraception was inadvisable because of other medication which the young woman was taking, and an intrauterine device was considered impracticable. As we shall see below, enforcing contraception, especially by injection, is itself invasive and requires careful consideration.

Mr Justice Bush in the High Court gave leave to Sunderland for sterilization. The Official Solicitor, as guardian *ad litem* for Jeanette, appealed. In the Court of Appeal Lord Justice Dillon said that the court had jurisdiction to authorize a sterilization on a ward of court, that it should only be as a last resort, but in this case, on the facts, it was appropriate.[3] He stated clearly that a natural parent or local authority with parental rights could not give consent to sterilization without first obtaining the leave of the court. A further appeal to the House of Lords was allowed, which, as we have seen, agreed with both lower courts.

The 'Jeanette' case raises a number of awkward questions: on what criteria should sterilization be undertaken on a mentally handicapped person deemed incompetent; what test is used for competency; and what jurisdiction do the courts have in respect of an incompetent adult (that is, someone over the age of 18). The first of these questions raises the ethical and moral issues inherent in treating any person without his or her consent; the second raises both ethical and practical issues of determining competency; and the third brings with it a complex discussion of Crown prerogative, common law, and the possible need for legislation to clarify the legal position.

Before proceeding to address these questions it is important to establish the sorts of persons with which this discussion is concerned. Many of the ethical and legal issues are relevant to persons other than those with mental handicap – people with severe mental illnesses or elderly mentally infirm people, for example, may, at some time, be unable to understand the nature of, and reason for, treatment. However, our concern here is only for those categorized as 'mentally handicapped'.

However mental handicap is a broad and ill-defined term. It has been described as 'arrested or incomplete development of mind',[4] a defect of intellectual functioning often due to congenital abnormality or inheritable condition, sometimes associated with prenatal trauma and occasionally serious accident or illness in childhood or later life. The American Association on Mental Deficiency defined mental deficiency (mental handicap) as 'significantly sub-average intellectual functioning which manifests itself during the developmental period and is characterised by inadequacy in adaptive behaviour'.

For the purposes of this discussion, mental handicap does not include progressive disorders such as Alzheimers Disease or brain damage due to alcohol abuse, even though the effects may, by and large, be the same. However, a further confusion arises because the terminology is constantly changing. The term 'mental deficiency' (Mental Deficiency Act 1913) was replaced with 'mental retardation' (still current in the USA) and eventually in the 1950s by 'mental handicap'. Recently, people with mental handicaps and their advocates have begun to use the term 'learning difficulty'. Although such a term implies social and education needs, and removes the stigma of a 'mental' (and overtly medical) label, it is nonetheless somewhat confusing. Many people have learning difficulties who do not have a mental handicap. Whilst respecting the wishes of people with mental handicap (or learning difficulties), we do need a commonly understood term.

The term 'mental handicap' will be used throughout this discussion, and should be understood as an intellectual disability of varying degrees. The terms 'profound', 'severe', 'moderate', and 'mild' mental handicap are to be avoided as predisposing certain attitudes and thus treatment. In any event no clear boundaries exist between these descriptions, and attempts to attach IQ levels or chronological age equivalents are fraught with problems. It is worth noting that mental handicap is highly variable, from those with very substantial handicap and minimal intellectual functioning to those with only minor educational disability (until recently, often referred to as mildly educationally subnormal). This discussion is concerned with those in the grey area between competency to understand and take decisions about the nature and purpose of some act (either to be done to them or by them) and those who, on any objective test, are not competent to take decisions for themselves. It is this distinction which is crucial. Even if a person is not competent, of course, this does not obviate the need for clear ethical criteria if any invasive (or 'touch') treatment is contemplated.

The ethical issues

The variable nature of mental handicap challenges fundamental ethical concepts. In particular the autonomy – paternalism conflict is brought into sharp relief. A hundred years ago paternalism held sway. Mentally handicapped people were kept out of harm's way in institutions or workhouses. Many died in infancy, and for some disorders, such as Down's syndrome, life expectancy was short. Various authors of that time mention people with mental handicaps, usually in less than complimentary ways.[5] Moreover, the mentally handicapped were amongst those groups seen as vulnerable to involuntary sterilization programmes instituted in the earlier part of this century in, for example, the USA. As people deemed 'unfit for parenting' their right to reproduce was systematically removed.[6]

Since the Second World War attitudes have begun to change. Generally, people with mental handicaps have been treated primarily as people with their disability as a secondary consideration. Their autonomy is seen as important and they are properly given every assistance to act independently with appropriate help and support. The self-advocacy movement is one manifestation of this new-found freedom of expression and the desire of the mentally handicapped to be considered seriously as equal citizens.

For some, autonomy is impaired by the severity of their handicap. A person may be capable of the day-to-day actions of an independent life – cooking, cleaning, washing, shopping – but still require help in dealing with money, or with more complicated matters such as legal contracts. Another person may be more handicapped and able to undertake simple tasks unaided but only in a fully supportive environment. His or her autonomy to undertake these tasks, to make friends, pursue leisure activities and so on must be respected; but regular paternalistic intervention occurs. At some level of disability paternalistic intervention becomes dominant and controlling, usually explained as being in the best interests of the handicapped person.

Unfortunately, the needs (and wants) of parents and carers sometimes intrude. Disentangling the best interests of the handicapped person independently from the best interests of the overall situation can be both difficult and stressful for all concerned. Sterilization is only the most emotive of a number of invasive procedures which require consent from the handicapped person, or in the absence of competent consent, very careful consideration of that person's needs.

Decisions may have to be taken on behalf of a person with mental handicap in relation to mental or physical health care (abortion, sterilization, hysterectomy, epilepsy, gynaecological examination, contraception), and concern about sexual or physical abuse (particularly of non-competent adults), legal contract, or social matters such as housing, education and day-to-day money matters. Although all of these may require paternalistic intervention it is not normal to see the High Court brought into decisions about, for example, a residential or school placement. Health (especially anything of doubtful therapeutic value) and money are the two areas which generate the most contention. Legal and monetary issues have their own mechanisms through the Court of Protection; health-related matters have no specific forum for resolution.

The reason may be found in the reversibility (or otherwise) of a decision. By and large social decisions – education, housing, leisure – are reversible. Health decisions – and, often, financial decisions – are not. Once the uterus is removed, or the money spent, it is gone. In addition, sterilization and abortion (and any similar procedures including contraception) are highly emotive. Both are invasive and (usually) irreversible; both are concerned with life in a fundamental way; and both strike at the root of one of the most powerful drives of human beings – the right, or at least desire, to procreate. No-one lightly gives up that ability. Nor do such concerns only affect women. Too often the discussion turns on sterilization of the woman and little or no thought is given to the possible sterilization of men. Whilst it is a truism that it is women who become pregnant, nonetheless much of the recent debate has been sexist. The simple assumption has been made that it is the woman's problem and there is nothing that men can do either to ease the problem, or to see it as affecting both sexes. Sterilization of all the men who might come into contact with Jeanette might seem extreme, but such a notion did not even enter the debate. It remains true that one of the major reasons for sterilization often given by parents – that it will widen the freedom of the woman concerned – would be equally valid if all men that were likely to have sexual intercourse with that woman were considered for sterilization – perhaps all those at the hostel or day centre. Such a step is not seriously canvassed here, but is raised to demonstrate the one-sided nature of the discussion.

Sterilization, then, is a particularly emotive issue. Many non-handicapped women consent to sterilization every year, usually as a permanent contraceptive device where therapeutic reasons are not overwhelming. Presumably those women discuss the matter with a competent gynaecologist and, if he or she agrees, there is no further legal difficulty. Sometimes the woman will be referred for counselling if the doctor is not convinced that the woman has given sufficient consideration to the consequences. However, unless the woman is seriously mentally ill or handicapped her wish will be accepted. Thus, the woman's autonomy is respected. Sterilization is

> . . . an operation of sufficient potential benefit and sufficiently small likely harm to be justified if a patient understandingly and autonomously agrees to it, and there are no generally overriding considerations of justice either in terms of people's rights or in terms of distribution of resources to prevent such operations.[7]

Difficulties arise when a person is not competent to take independent decisions – that is, when their autonomy is in question, either because:

1 he/she has lost a previous ability to act autonomously (for example, a comatose patient found at the scene of a road accident);
2 he/she has not reached the point at which it is conceded that autonomous behaviour is possible (for example, small children); or
3 he/she has never been able to act autonomously (for example a severely intellectually disabled person).

In the first case the usual procedure is to look back to when the person was able to act autonomously and to try to decide how he/she would have acted. This is not always possible and is sometimes unhelpful. In the second case proxy consent is usually given by parents who are assumed to be acting in the child's best interests, unless this can be proved otherwise. Often health professionals will override a parent's religious beliefs if detrimental to the child, until age 18 (in Britain) when the person is deemed capable of voluntarily espousing such beliefs.

The third case is the most difficult. There is no previous autonomous history, yet treating the person as a child belies the true nature of their disability; and once over 18, proxy consent has no validity. People with mental handicaps have complex personalities like everyone else. To talk of a mental age or two or three is meaningless. Although intellectually he/she may only function at that level, life skills may approximate to those of a child of five or six (or eight or nine) and, socially, the person may be capable of adolescent or adult interaction. Often, too, a person may not be capable of much academically but can have a good grasp of their own interests, especially their personal body integrity. Consequently, any decision on sterilization, or similar procedures, must be taken carefully. The 'bottom line' is that any decision taken must not harm the person's interests. A preferable view is that it is *in* his or her interests; the most preferable that it is in his or her *best* interests.

A number of questions are, however, raised by the use of this language: for example, what are those interests? when is a person not competent? and who should make decisions on the person's behalf? We shall see below the different procedures for those below and above the age of 18, and the role of the court in making judgements. At this point, however, it should be noted that competency is always assumed unless it is shown otherwise.

The validity of allowing sterilization can be considered in two ways. The first suggests that proxy consent to sterilization is not acceptable because:

1 it is never in the person's interests;
2 it violates the person's rights;
3 it is against society's interests.

Such an approach places us in the position of opposing sterilization on anything but a truly voluntary basis; and any discussion will tend towards allowing sterilization. Conversely, this can be turned on its head, and the arguments made by those who would allow sterilization can then be examined on the basis of proxy consent on the grounds that:

(i) it is broadly in society's interests to allow sterilization of handicapped people;
(ii) far from violating a right to reproduce there is a right to freedom of social and sexual expression – or sometimes put more succinctly that it does not violate any 'rights' because the person is incapable of exercising those rights; and
(iii) it is in the best interests of the person.

This latter set of arguments will be taken as a basis for this discussion as it requires us to analyse widely held views and to focus initially on the major reasons advanced for sterilization.

The 'interests of society' argument is essentially utilitarian; as a rule 'the happiness of the greatest number' (of both mentally handicapped people and the general population) will be served by sterilizing some severely handicapped people. Several reasons are advanced. In the first place it is assumed that a mentally handicapped woman will be unable to care for her child and it will become a burden on society. Even if one ignores the contentious suggestion that people, by virtue of being handicapped, *will* be unable to look after their children properly, it is not inevitable that

– in cases where this does turn out to be true – this is the only available option. In fact in Britain at present there are too few babies available relative to the number of couples eager to adopt. Whilst this cannot possibly sustain an argument for *encouraging* mentally handicapped women to have children, the small number of likely births cannot be considered a serious burden on the state. Nor can it justify the radical invasion of fundamental civil liberties which its routine acceptance would predict.

More pressing as an argument might be the burden on parents, some of whom in the past have themselves adopted their daughters' children. This does indeed arise as an argument for sterilization. Carers often look after handicapped sons and daughters with little help in cash or kind – welfare income benefits or services. Dealing with menstruation can be difficult; constant vigilance in social relations can be tiring if not impossible. But is the convenience of relatives really an acceptable argument for an irreversible step such as sterilization? The court in the Canadian case of *Re Eve*[8] were in no doubt that human rights could not be invaded because of the potential impact on a third party – in this case the mother of 'Eve' – however much sympathy she merited.

Third, some handicapping conditions are inheritable. The competent woman will often decide not to have children, or, after genetic counselling, take a calculated risk. If a handicapped foetus is produced, abortion would most probably be the chosen treatment, not sterilization. Sterilization would only be routinely indicated where a dominant gene gives rise to a high risk at each pregnancy of a severely handicapped child. The same balance of considerations should apply to mentally handicapped women. Unfortunately, sterilization for these reasons runs the risk of escaping the very narrow confines for which it is intended, and becoming a general eugenic programme.

Here we come to the 'slippery slope'. At what level of handicap do we decide a woman is incapable of looking after a child, or should be *required* to have a (eugenic?) sterilization or abortion? And who decides? 'Slippery slope' arguments are generally thought not to be good philosophy. They are of two sorts – logical and empirical. Logically there is no clear line of argument from the difficulties (and needs) of some mentally handicapped women and those of ordinary women. If sterilization is only ever done in the best interests of the person concerned, the dangers of mass eugenic programmes are too remote to be given serious consideration. Unfortunately, we cannot be so sanguine about the empirical slope. Observed attitudes suggest that allowing sterilization on the basis of anything but the most stringent criteria will lead to demands by some for the sterilization of competent handicapped or non-handicapped women. Recent work on the Third Reich has demon-strated the connection between early sterilization programmes on handicapped people and the later mass murders and medical exper-imentation in places such as Auschwitz.[9] The moral hygiene move-ment in the USA and Germany in the early part of the century was supported by many eminent doctors. From there to equating biological with social pathology was a relatively easy step; and social pathology could be erased by cutting out the 'diseased part' of the social body. In Germany in the 1930s that diseased part was the non-Aryan minorities – particularly the Jews. We must always be on our guard against this sort of distorted 'logic'. For example, compulsory sterilization of HIV-infected intravenous drug users has already been suggested. Wider acceptance of sterilization would certainly raise expectations amongst parents that their caring prob-lems could be reduced. It is thus not in society's interests to allow sterilization except under strict controls. Careful consideration against clear guidelines should be given to each case.

The second of the threefold reasons for proxy consent is the argument about rights. In the case of *Re D (a minor)*[10] Mrs Justice Heilbron said:

> . . . sterilisation is an operation which involves the deprivation of a basic human right, namely the right of a woman to reproduce, and therefore it would if performed on a woman for non-therapeutic reasons and without her consent be a violation of that right.[11]

The case before the court in that instance was concerned with wardship proceedings for the purpose of sterilizing a 10 year-old girl with Sotos syndrome. 'D' was mentally handicapped and epileptic, though her handicap was relatively mild. The court took the view that she would be able to continue to learn and might attain sufficient understanding to be able to marry and have children. More important in this case were the conditions of severe depri-vation in which the family lived and which were largely the reasons for the mother asking for sterilization to be performed. In summary Mrs Justice Heilbron stated:

> A review of the whole of the evidence leads me to the conclusion that in the case of a child of 11 years of age where the evidence shows that her mental and physical conditions and attainments have already improved and where her future prospects are as yet unpre-dictable, where the evidence also shows that she is unable *as yet* to understand and appreciate the implications of this operation and could not give valid or informed consent, but the likelihood that in later years she will be able to make her own choice, where I believe the frustration and resentment of realising (as she would one day)

what had happened, could be devastating, an operation of this nature is in my view, contra-indicated.[12]

Some have claimed that the right to reproduce is only a right if the person is able to claim or enforce that right. Others may accept that there is a right of sorts, but might question whether or not it is a fundamental right; or could it be defensible, as in China, where, in consideration of society's resources, each couple may legally have only one child? If there is a right to reproduce is there a converse right *not* to have to reproduce – for example, if a person is unable to give a meaningful or valid consent to sexual intercourse or has no understanding of the potential outcome of their act?

Rights, simply, are natural or legal. In the case of natural (or, for our purposes, human) rights, the person has that right by virtue of his or her status as a human being. Legal rights are conferred on those persons who are citizens (or come under the jurisdiction) of a particular legal authority. In either case, rights cannot simply be taken away. As there is no law either expressly allowing or expressly forbidding reproduction, the right can be considered a derivative human right rooted in the right to life and freedom from arbitrary interference. A human right is something which a person has regardless of whether, for some reason, at some time, that person is unable autonomously to claim, enforce or waive that right. Babies are human persons but cannot, at that stage in their lives, autonomously enforce their rights. Nonetheless, by extrapolation, we can extend ordinary rights to babies as human persons. Given their rights they will grow to be autonomous rights holders. This remains true even if the person grows to have only limited autonomy: he or she remains a human person on the usual spectrum of human ability. If we extend rights to the non-handicapped baby (who will grow to be a non-handicapped adult) then we must also extend those rights to the non-autonomous adult. We must conclude, therefore, that if reproduction is a right then mentally handicapped women cannot lose that right simply by virtue of their mental handicap.

However, rights can come into conflict. With some validity a claim may be made that if a person:

(a) cannot understand the connection between sexual intercourse and pregnancy,
(b) may find pregnancy and childbirth traumatic,
(c) could not possibly look after any child produced, and
(d) is likely to have sexual relations unless confined continually.

then paternalistically there is a right *not* to reproduce – that is, that people should be protected from reproducing by removal of their capacity to do so.

It is instructive at this point to consider social attitudes about fertility. How many women would willingly give up control over their fertility and return to the days before the availability of contraception, with the possibility of having a dozen children in as many years? Some, yes, by consent. Most, no! The right to reproduce includes a right to control fertility on the grounds of health, personal lifestyle (including career options) and economics. A non-competent woman should be subject to similar considerations. There can be no absolute violation of the right to reproduce if the 'transgression' of that right follows a conflict of rights and is decided in the best interests of the individual. We must be suspicious, though, of the convenience of carers dressed up as a 'right to wider freedoms'. Any conflicting right must be carefully analysed as to its applicability in the specific instance.

The last of the three arguments outlined above is the 'best interests' test. Sterilization for entirely therapeutic reasons (because of a cancerous uterus, for example) is clearly in the best interests of that person. Indeed, on the principle of double effect, sterilization is merely the inevitable (even if undesirable) consequence of a 'good' act – that is, saving the life of the woman concerned. Few, if any, would object to proxy consent for such a life-saving treatment. On the other hand, most, if not all, would draw the line at enforcing a non-therapeutic, though non-life threatening procedure, even if a great benefit would accrue to some third party. For example, consider the case of a non-competent mentally handicapped woman asked to give one of her kidneys to assist her brother in end-stage renal failure. All would agree that, in the absence of informed consent, there is no right to remove that organ even though the brother will die without it (and the woman would continue to live with only one kidney). It is not in her interests at all, certainly not her best interests, to lose a kidney. The best interests test must relate *only* to the person in question.

However, the distinction often used in such situations is that the intervention is therapeutic rather than non-therapeutic, thus – in theory at least – enhancing the possibility of proxy consent being held to be valid. Therapeutic intervention is generally that which is undertaken to benefit the individual concerned and not other members of the community. The assumption, therefore, is that the intervention will resolve a medical condition of the individual rather than enhancing the social conditions of that person's carers. Yet, unless courts are very careful, medical acts which *are* designed primarily to avoid social difficulties can be forced into the framework of 'therapeutic' treatment. A number of recent decisions[13] have shown that courts may – however unwittingly – slip into a pattern of decision-making which blurs this important destinction. For example, in *In Matter of Sallmaier*,[14] no clear distinction was drawn between therapeutic and non-therapeutic intervention.

On the other hand, in the case of *Re 'Eve'*[15] the Canadian court recognized the proposed sterilization as being 'admittedly non-therapeutic' and concluded on evidence from other court decisions that there was a real danger of using non-therapeutic grounds as if they were therapeutic in order to serve what the court wished to identify as the 'best interests' of the person. They referred, for example, to the case of *Re K*,[16] in which a British Columbia court ordered that a hysterectomy could be carried out on a retarded child on the basis of her alleged phobic reaction to blood, which it was thought might pose serious problems should she be permitted to commence menstruation. Although the court was at pains to say that ' . . . this case cannot and must not be regarded as a precedent to be followed in cases involving sterilization of mentally handicapped persons for contraceptive purposes'[17] the 'slippery slope' argument outlined above cannot be entirely dismissed as having no influence on subsequent courts. Once the principle of radical intrusion is conceded on grounds which are somewhat dubious, there is no telling where it might end.

Of course, a further question remains, and that is: can non-voluntary sterilization ever be in a person's interests? We must presume the non-consenting, non-competent woman will have similar wants and needs to the ordinary woman. Normally sterilization without consent for therapeutic or non-therapeutic reasons would be regarded as a gross intrusion. Sterilization is undertaken by some women solely to escape pregnancy – usually, but not exclusively, as a foolproof contraceptive measure after having a family. Sterilization is unlikely, however, to be the treatment of choice for monthly period cramps or because the management of heavy menstruation may be messy.[18] The psychological value of the ability to bear children is of enormous importance and dictates the informed choice.

Sterilization requires surgical intervention, probably under a general anaesthetic. Yet such risks are taken by ordinary women daily. The procedure (rather than the reasons for it or its outcome) cannot, of itself, therefore, be a reason for not sterilizing a woman.[19] Nonetheless it is widely accepted that it may be beneficial – even the treatment of choice – to be sterilized. If so, mentally handicapped women should have the same choices, as far as possible.

Opponents of non-consenting sterilization argue that it should only be undertaken under very extreme circumstances. At the same time, they will argue that care should be taken to ensure the woman does not become pregnant. Indeed this subject is fraught with potential double standards of that sort. Where it is possible to teach the person with mental handicap to use a barrier method of contraception – a condom or cap – the only issue is the degree of paternalism which can be justified. Unfortunately many of those with whom we are concerned here are unlikely to be able to understand how such devices are to be used even following detailed and elaborate training. Such training may also be distasteful to parents and perceived as encouraging sexual intercourse. But if training and education were given to *all* mentally handicapped men in clubs, hostels and institutions in using condoms – which were then freely available – many of these problems would disappear. Certainly a moral irony is apparent. Some parents and guardians are content to permit an invasive, irreversible procedure – sometimes on a woman capable of understanding or growing to understanding pregnancy (as in *Re D*[20]) – yet object to explicit sex education and contraceptive advice, although research has demonstrated that women with mental handicaps can be taught to say 'no'.[21]

Although long-acting injectible contraceptives (for example, depoprovera) or oral contraceptive pills are invasive procedures requiring consent, at least they have the benefit of reversibility. No final decision is taken and it can be reviewed regularly as a person develops. The question of reversibility is important in an assessment of appropriate intervention, although some have argued that it is no more than a red herring. Equally, the implications of reversible techniques must be taken into account. If a woman is never likely to grow to understand, the contraceptive may have to be given for the whole of the woman's fertile life. As contraceptive drugs are implicated in various disorders, and intrauterine devices in, amongst other things, heavy, irregular bleeding, long-term use may not be medically in the person's best interests. Sterilization, in this situation, is both therapeutic and gives greater freedom of sexual activity and physical well-being. Even so, it must be said that only where irreversibility can be shown to be wholly irrelevant should sterilization be considered.

In summary, the ethical arguments demonstrate that sterilization without the consent of the handicapped person is not entirely or inevitably unacceptable, but suggest that it must be used only when:

(a)   it is in the best interests of the woman concerned, and
(b)   no other reversible contraceptive device is acceptable for good medical or therapeutic reasons; or
(c)   it can be shown that irreversibility is wholly irrelevant to the woman's needs, and never solely (or even largely) because

of the convenience of carers, or a simple lack of capacity to consent.

So far, the best interests test has turned on:

1   the much greater freedom of the woman to have social and sexual relations unhindered by the prospect of pregnancy;
2   the likelihood that pregnancy itself would be traumatic or dangerous to the woman's health; and
3   that the woman could not possibly understand the nature of childbirth or look after the child produced.

The last point is contentious. Whilst there must be no suggestion of encouraging handicapped women to have unwanted babies, the state can provide for such children. If all the logical and empirical dangers flow only from concern about a very few unwanted children, then this is not in itself a sufficient or reasonable ground for allowing non-voluntary sterilization. The first point is also somewhat contentious, except if a rigorous rights-based analysis, similar to that described here, is applied – and even then only in extreme cases. Except for those cases, only (2) above is strictly concerned with the woman's best interests. Care must be taken to avoid the importation of other considerations, such as the social or eugenic, since these offer dangerous potential for the future.

We turn now to the legal issues. In the final section a proposal is offered for the stringent conditions on which sterilization could be allowed on the non-consenting child or adult.

Legal aspects

The legal issues turn on competency – the ability or otherwise to make an informed judgement of proposed procedures. Those concerned with sterilizing mentally handicapped people will argue that the handicapped person is not competent to make such judgements: proxy consent is therefore required and is acceptable, since otherwise no intervention could go ahead. Severely mentally handicapped people, it is argued, do not understand sexual intercourse and pregnancy, the nature and purpose of contraception, the nature of childbirth and childcare, nor the procedure of sterilization. In their best interests, proxy consent should be given for sterilization without (but not inevitably against) the person's own consent. On the assumption of best interests, when is the person deemed not competent?

Unfortunately there is no legal definition of competency. Various

UK statutes define circumstances when a person can be treated against his or her will. In particular, the Mental Health Act 1983 (1984 in Scotland) enables treatment to be given when a person ' . . . ought to be detained in the interests of his own health or safety or with a view to the protection of other persons'. Competency is not mentioned, only implied. Sections 57 and 58 of the same Act enable the patient to consent to treatment under certain conditions whilst detained unless 'a registered medical practitioner . . . has certified in writing that the patient is not capable of understanding the nature, purpose and likely effects of treatment'.[22] Competency to consent is not defined, although the clause itself could be deemed a test of competency for the purposes of the Act.

Although the Statute does not apply to mentally handicapped people (except those very few who come within the ambit of mental impairment or severe mental impairment) the paucity of definition is demonstrated. At the same time, it offers some boundaries to treatment on those deemed not capable of consent. For example the 1978 White Paper[23] suggested that where a patient's consent was not forthcoming (either due to non-competency, or competent opposition) the responsible consultant (that is, doctor) should 'wherever there is a choice, select the method of treatment the patient finds least objectionable or which represents the minimum interference with the patient'.[24]

A similar philosophy ought to inform our concerns here. Competency is a variable commodity. Every person is more or less competent at undertaking differing tasks. The neurosurgeon may be competent to give an informed view of a neurological complication, but not willing to risk an opinion in some other branch of medicine, let alone a problem of civil engineering. Competency hinges on more than intellectual ability. Education, prior knowledge and experience are all important. Where intellectual capacity is impaired, such factors take on greater emphasis. Competency can be enhanced by care, resources to aid understanding, as well as information delivered in accessible ways. Competency is often not located wholly in the individual but can be, and often is, shared. For our purposes, competency turns on the understanding of choice. Competency is thus context-related and dynamic and requires sufficient ability to understand that a decision on options is required. Any decision on competency must be seen to be reasonable using tests sympathetic to the nature of mental handicap and the widely divergent levels of understanding unrelated directly to educational ability or attainment. Competency could therefore be defined along the following lines: to arrive at a decision on a particular procedure (for example, sterilization) a test based on reasonableness must be applied to ascertain if the person has sufficient understanding

(a) that there is a choice to be made;
(b) of the proposed action to be taken, and its consequential benefits and risks.

Such a definition would help parents, professionals and courts. Decisions on the reasonable test of 'sufficient understanding' need to be made by a multidisciplinary group and not by a sole professional acting alone. After all, even lack of competency does not allow non-therapeutic procedures unless they can be shown to be in the person's best interests. Even where a person is not competent there must still be recourse to the courts to enable the sanctioning of such procedures as sterilization.[25]

Wardship jurisdiction is needed because (a) the court must satisfy itself as to the best interests of the child (and as we shall see later, the adult), and (b) it protects those carrying out the procedure. Common law is clear that:

1 any form of physically invasive treatment applied without consent is a battery – a wrong against the physical person; and
2 a patient's consent should be real – that is, genuine – uninfluenced by coercion, fraud or misdescription, and informed; and
3 any person proposing treatment is under a duty to use reasonable care and skill.

Although a non-competent person may have great difficulty in briefing advocates to bring a case of battery, nonetheless the official solicitor or other *guardian ad litem* could bring an action in damages. Sanction is therefore usually sought – especially following the judgement in *Re B*,[26] and in line with the United Nations Declaration of Rights for the Mentally Handicapped Person.[27]

Proxy consent is allowed in law on behalf of minors, usually by parents or guardians such as local authorities, or more rarely through wardship in the High Court (in England and Wales). The judgement in the Gillick case,[28] which dealt with the provision of contraceptive advice to girls under 16 suggested that the need for proxy consent declines in importance the nearer a competent person is to the age of 18.[29] It was also held that, although it was unlawful for a man to have sexual intercourse with a girl under 16, nonetheless contraceptive advice could be given.[30] A person over 16 may give full consent – for example to surgical intervention – [31] although some have suggested that this may be overridden by parents. Scottish law takes the position that there is no presumption that children under the age of 16 are incompetent to give consent. This is partially based on a commonsense approach to the differing levels of maturity of children, and partly on the Scottish law division of children into pupils (boys under 14 and girls under 12) and minors.[32] Over the age of majority no other person can give consent on behalf of that person, however disabled.

The first legal problem is thus the nature and extent of competency. The second has been highlighted by *In Re B*[33] in England, and *Re 'Eve'*[34] in Canada: that is, the question as to whether the courts have jurisdiction to order or allow any procedure on a non-competent adult. Some commentators argue there is strictly no power, others that it exists under the ancient *parens patriae* powers of the Crown. Wardship is just a special case and one with a clear aetiology and use. The *Re B*[35] case highlighted this problem forcefully. As was noted earlier 'B' (Jeanette) was 17 when Sunderland Borough Council brought wardship proceedings. She was already in care, but with unseemly haste her case was heard first in the High Court, then the Court of Appeal and eventually the House of Lords gave judgement just 20 days before her eighteenth birthday. A few days' delay would theoretically have precluded any action. Wardship is usually sought (normally by a local authority) to protect a minor, often from its own parents. In B's case this can be understood if it is assumed that Sunderland were acting in B's interests. Some would say they were not, the eventual judgement notwithstanding, and the action was more in the carers' interests than B's.

Although the ward's interests have in recent years assumed prominence, it was not always so. Wardship history is confused and proceedings have been brought in both the wards' and guardians' interests. *Parens patriae* (literally 'father of the people') and wardship derive from separate sources. Speculatively, *parens patriae* stems from the late thirteenth century or early fourteenth century when '[B]y general assent or by some statute, now lost, the care of persons of unsound mind was by Edward I taken from the feudal lords, who would naturally take possession of the land of a tenant unable to perform his feudal duties'.[36]

Wardship, on the other hand, arose from property rights arising out of feudal tenures, and was originally intended to protect the rights of the guardian. Over time, wardship became 'substantively and procedurally assimiliated to parens patriae, lost the connection with property and became purely protective in nature. Wardship thus is . . . a device . . . [to] . . . exercise [the] parens patriae jurisdiction [over children].'[37]

Apart from the Mental Health Act, certain other statutes allow for removal of those competent to care for themselves but do not provide for treatment without consent. Common law allows for emergency treatment if there is an immediate or present serious danger to the life or health of the person.[38] Sometimes treatment is given in the absence of emergency, especially in psychiatry, on the 'thank you' principle – that when the person is recovered they will be grateful for the intervention. A better term is 'implied consent', which is, however, ethically suspect. Implied consent is always a fiction and in some cases is clearly counterfactual – such as in treating the unconscious person who has attempted suicide. Nonetheless one formulation which is to some extent based on what a person might have consented to, if competent, is given by Culver and Gert.[39] They offer a useful approach to paternalistic intervention which can be adapted for our purposes: sterilization is only justified if:

1 the amount of evil probably prevented or ameliorated for the woman is very great;
2 the amount of evil perpetrated on the woman by sterilization is so much less than the evil probably prevented that it would have been irrational of her, if able to consent, to have preferred not to be sterilized; and
3 there is no other known adequate reason (for example, religious or political) for not undertaking sterilization.

Deciding on the balance of evils (or harms) is difficult, although such a formula cautions us to be exceedingly rigorous in considering the interests of the woman. Doctors and other professionals are understandably becoming wary about the doctrine of 'implied consent' or 'necessity'. Neither may be watertight, and challenges from civil rights advocates demand firmer ground.

Consequently, a way forward (proposed by Kennedy[40] amongst others) is to re-establish *parens patriae* jurisdiction for adults. Considerable impetus had been given to this proposal by a learned and carefully researched judgement by LaForest in the 'Eve' case in Canada.[41] Although Canadian law differs from English or Scottish law, it is rooted in the same history (especially English law). In particular, the Chancery Act appears to give some jurisdiction to the Lord Chancellor (in England) over 'mentally handicapped' persons. For example, in the fairly recent case of *Re X (a minor)* [42] Mr Justice Latey, dealing with a 14 year-old girl, said ' . . . I can find nothing in the authorities . . . to suggest there is any limitation in the theoretical scope of this jurisdiction'.[43] Although this case concerned a minor, the point is that it can be said that wardship, as procedurally similar to *parens patriae*, is 'of the widest nature' and not limited by precedent.

Earlier judgements have suggested that those limits which do exist depend on circumstances and that the courts can act to protect non-competent mentally handicapped people. The power, as Lord Eldon put it ' . . . belongs to the King as parens patriae . . . and is founded on the obvious necessity that the law should place somewhere the care of individuals who cannot take care of themselves.'[44]

Whether this power is available to an English court is another matter. Statute may have replaced common law and thereby abolished the power. Whatever the position with common law, the power was lost on the enactment of the Mental Health Act 1959. In that Act, it is argued, the Crown prerogative was expressly removed. Kennedy argues that the *express* removal is unsustainable, by simple inspection of the wording of the Act. However, removal by necessary implication is possible, although the courts are reluctant to accept this unless it is *truly* necessary. In this case, only property affairs are covered (by s. 95(1) of the 1983 Mental Health Act (England and Wales)). Treatment decisions are *not* covered and could be said not to be affected by those Acts.

Kennedy cites a further complication. The guardianship provisions of the Mental Health Act 1959 specifically conferred on a guardian all the power exercisable in law by a father of a child under 14 (s. 34(1)). However, most mentally handicapped people were removed from the 1983 Act, including the guardianship powers (ironically an omission much lamented by parents and mental handicap organizations). The removal of mentally handicapped people from the Act could be said to restore the guardianship powers under *parens patriae* which had been superseded by the 1959 Act. Another way of looking at it is to say that the prerogative power was in abeyance and is now extant again. Alternatively it could be argued that, with the loss of guardianship from the 1983 Act, no one now has the power or right to consent for a mentally handicapped adult. On balance, Kennedy argues that the power is available, on the grounds that constitutional theory does not like the abolition of a prerogative power but can accept a period of abeyance. The Crown, perhaps, cannot tolerate a vacuum.

In the 'Eve' case the court decided it did have the power to order a sterilization but only where the procedure was therapeutic. Even so, the court was not prepared to order sterilization of 'Eve' as it considered this would not be on her best interests. Moreover, the court took serious account of the conclusion of the Law Commission of Canada that:

> . . . like anyone else, the mentally handicapped have individually varying reactions to sterilization. Sex and parenthood hold the same significance for them as for other people and their misconceptions

and misunderstandings are also similar. The psychological impact of sterilization is likely to be particularly damaging in cases where it is a result of coercion and when the mentally handicapped have had no children.[45]

'Eve' was in her twenties – an attractive young woman. Although it was agreed that caring for any child produced would probably be beyond her, she was quite capable of understanding the nature of sexual relations. Indeed, it was the presence of a steady boyfriend that had encouraged the mother to bring the action. In giving judgement Mr Justice La Forest said:

> The grave intrusion on a person's rights and the certain physical damage that ensues from non-therapeutic sterilisation without consent, when compared to the highly questionable advantages that can result from it, have persuaded me that it can never safely be determined that such a procedure is for the benefit of the person. Accordingly the procedure should never be authorised for non-therapeutic purposes under the parens patriae jurisdiction.[46]

Nor was Mr Justice La Forest prepared to follow an often-canvassed route different from the 'best interests' test – namely the 'substituted judgement' test. Under this kind of analysis, as with the suicide example mentioned above, the court could opt to presume that, had the person been competent to choose, then they would have chosen sterilization. As Mr Justice La Forest said:

> . . . it is obviously fiction to suggest that a decision so made is that of the mental incompetent. What the incompetent would do if he or she could make the choice is simply a matter of speculation.[47]

Even if the courts have power to order a sterilization on a non-competent adult, the question of procedure still arises. Too many decisions are taken on an *ad hoc* basis with little reference to guiding principles; and in any event the courts ought to be a last resort. Some form of local ethical committees might be a better option, with a set of guidelines established nationally. Any local dissent could be referred to a tribunal, and only in rare cases to the High Court, although resort to a court must always be an option in accordance with the United Nations agreement referred to above.[48] Consistency, as an aspect of formal justice, is an important concomitant of a morally acceptable approach, and removing as much variability from professional or court decisions as possible requires guiding principles to be set by a competent national body such as the Law Commission. We have seen, however, how difficult and contentious the formulation of those principles might be. There is no easy solution and, to a degree, each case may have to be judged on its merits.

Conclusions

In essence, a review of the problems, from both a philosophical and a practical viewpoint, suggests that it must be concluded that it is impossible to say that sterilization of a non-competent minor or adult will *never* be in the person's best interests. We *can* say it should be undertaken only rarely and after careful consideration of the facts; and we can assert that the criteria adopted should be narrow and distinct, and ones which minimize the likelihood of slippery slopes. However, given that no criteria can be hard and fast or fully objective, a grey area will still exist. Any compromise demanded in the interest of public policy must understand and take seriously the true needs of the severely handicapped person even whilst recognizing the serious public issues involved.

Instead of a slippery slope we need a narrow ledge with as vertical a cut-off as is possible. That 'ledge' will be defined by criteria which are inevitably somewhat subjective but simultaneously tight. The cut-off will not be vertical but is bound to be a slope of some sort. That slope must be as steep as possible to minimize the possibility that policy will creep down it. From the earlier discussion, the following criteria can tentatively be postulated. Sterilization can only be undertaken on a minor or adult without a competent consent when:

(a) it is in the best interests of the woman, based on the reasonable judgement of a multidisciplinary team, where the best interests are based on the likelihood that pregnancy would be dangerous to the woman's life or health; and

(b) no other reversible contraceptive device is acceptable for good medical or therapeutic reasons, and the woman is likely to have sexual relations which may lead to pregnancy.

If such criteria had been adopted in the *Re B* case,[49] it is still likely that sterilization would have been agreed. But this does no more than to reinforce the fact that this was an extreme case, and should not be used as an indicator of leniency towards sterilization or used to argue for its easier availability in such circumstances. Rather, the gravity of B's condition could be used to demonstrate that the *rule* must be no non-consensual sterilization, whilst exceptions require stringent and consistent justification on the lines suggested above.

As a final note, much of the discussion has been about steriliz-

ation of women. Few words have been said about men. The
necessity for a non-sexist debate and the potential for male sterilization and education on contraception have been noted. It remains
true, however, that it is women who are often left literally 'holding
the baby'. The criteria proposed are narrow and do not allow wide
interpretation. But we must not forget the individual woman, nor
her carers. Any solution to these problems must recognize the
urgent practical, personal and public issues and seek to be at once
compassionate and humanitarian.

Notes

1   In *Re B (a minor) (Sterilisation)* [1987] 2 All ER 206 (CA); *The Times*, 17 March
    1987 (HL)
2   Brahams, D., 'Court of Appeal agrees to sterilisation of 17-year-old mentally
    handicapped girl under wardship jurisdiction', *The Lancet*, 28 March 1987,
    pp. 757–8.
3   *Supra cit.*, note 1.
4   Mental Health Act 1959 (England and Wales); Mental Health (Scotland) Act
    1960.
5   See, for example, Charlotte Bronte's *Villette*.
6   For discussion, see Meyers, D., *The Human Body and the Law*, Edinburgh,
    University Press, 1971; McLean, S. A. M., 'The Right to Reproduce' in
    Campbell, T., Goldberg, D., McLean, S. A. M. and Mullen, T., (eds), *Human
    Rights: From Rhetoric to Reality*, Oxford, Basil Blackwell, 1986.
7   Gillon, R., 'On sterilising severely mentally handicapped people', **13** *Journal
    of Medical Ethics*, 1987, 59–61.
8   *Re 'Eve'* (1986) 2 SCR 407;
9   Lifton, R. J., *The Nazi Doctors*, New York, Macmillan, 1986.
10 *Re D (a minor)* [1976] 1 All ER 326.
11 Ibid., at p. 332.
12 Ibid., at p. 336.
13 Cf. *North Carolina Association for Retarded Children et al.* v. *State of North Carolina
    et al.* 420 F. Supp. 451 (1976).
14 *In matter of Sallmaier* (1976) 378 NYS 2d 989, where the court said, at p. 991:
    'The decision to exercise *parens patriae* must reflect the welfare of society as a
    whole, but mainly it must balance the individual's right to be free from
    interference against the individual's need to be treated, if treatment would in
    fact be in his best interest.'
15 *Supra cit.*, note 8.
16 *Re K* (1985) 19 DLR (4th) 255.
17 Ibid., at p. 275.
18 But see *Re K, supra cit.* note 16.
19 But see the now disregarded view of Lord Denning in *Bravery* v. *Bravery* [1954]
    3 All ER 59.
20 *Supra cit.*, note 10.
21 Cf. work undertaken by Prof. Peter Mittler, University of Manchester, Institute
    of Education.
22 Mental Health Act 1983; Jones, R. (ed.), *Mental Health Act Manual*, London,
    Sweet and Maxwell, 1985, pp. 109–11.

23 Cmnd 7320/1978
24 Ibid., para 6.18.
25 As noted by Mr Justice Wood (supported by Court of Appeal) in *Re B, supra cit.*, note 1.
26 See note 1, *supra.*
27 Charter of Rights for the Mentally Handicapped Person, adopted by the General Assembly of the United Nations, December 1971.
28 *Gillick* v. *North West Norfolk & Wisbech AHA & Anor* [1984] 1 All ER 365; [1985] 3 All ER 402; [1985] 3 All ER 830 (HL).
29 See also Lord Denning in *Hewer* v. *Bryant* [1969] 3 All ER 578, at p. 582.
30 *Gillick, supra cit.* note 28.
31 Family Law Reform Act 1969 s. 8.
32 For discussion, see Consultative Memorandum no. 65, *Legal Capacity and Responsibility of Minors and Pupils*, Scottish Law Commission, June 1985.
33 *Supra cit.*, note 1.
34 *Supra cit.*, note 8.
35 *Supra cit.*, note 1.
36 Theobald, H., *The Law Relating to Lunacy*, 1924, cited in *Re Eve*, note 8, *supra.*
37 *Re 'Eve' supra cit.* note 8.
38 Cf. Mason, J. K. and McCall Smith, R. A., *Law and Medical Ethics*, (2nd edn.), London, Butterworths, 1987.
39 Culver, C. M. and Gert, B., *Philosophy in Medicine*, New York/Oxford, Oxford University Press, 1982, at pp. 148 and 166.
40 Kennedy, I., Note to a conference organised by MENCAP/Royal Society of Medicine Section on Mental Retardation, 3–4 February 1988.
41 *Supra cit.*, note 8.
42 *Re X (a minor)* [1975] 1 All ER, 697.
43 Ibid., at p. 699.
44 In *Wellesley* v. *Duke of Beaufort* (1827) at 2 RUSS 18 38 ER 242.
45 Law Commission of Canada, *Sterilization*, Working Paper no. 24, 1979, at p. 50.
46 *Re 'Eve'*, note 8, *supra cit.*, at 390.
47 Note 8, *supra cit.*, at p. 435.
48 *Supra cit.*, note 27.
49 *Supra cit.*, note 1.

7 Is surrogacy exploitative?

MICHAEL FREEMAN

Introduction: the new folk devil

Surrogacy is a phenomenon which has burst on the scene in the 1980s,[1] causing a moral panic[2] in the UK, the first country to legislate[3] to control it, as well as a flurry of activity in other countries, with reports,[4] legislation[5] and a burgeoning of academic literature[6] and feminist critique.[7]

With infertility at new high levels of 10–15 per cent[8] and increasing,[9] with opportunities to adopt[10] healthy and acceptable[11] babies curtailed by relatively liberal abortion laws,[12] easier access to contraception[13] (in particular, the contraceptive pill) and greater toleration of single parenthood, it is difficult to see the demand for surrogacy (and other 'new ways of making babies')[14] diminishing. In the language of the economists, that demand is relatively inelastic. Probably no legal case in the world (the *Spycatcher* saga[15] apart) attracted greater worldwide attention in 1987 than 'Baby M',[16] and certainly there were few more controversial cases in Britain in 1986 than 'Baby Cotton'.[17]

Responses to surrogacy

Judicial responses to surrogacy have varied and, to some extent, mellowed. As Kleegan and Kaufman noted:

> Any change in custom or practice in this emotionally charged area has always elicited a response from established custom and law of horrified negation at first; then negation without horror; then slow and gradual curiosity, study, evaluation, and finally a very slow but steady acceptance.[18]

We are far from reaching the final stage yet, although there are

164

signs of it – particularly in the latest Ontario initiative,[19] But the other stages have all been seen. Compare the response of the Court of Appeal in the first surrogacy case in 1978[20] (at a time when the concept had not entered the vocabulary) to Mr Justice Latey's sympathy and tolerance in the 'Baby Cotton'[21] case or to his liberal willingness to assist the adopters of Kirsty Stevens's baby in a case decided in March 1987.[22] Similar patterns may be detected in the USA, where at first surrogacy agreements were frustrated[23] and latterly, in the Baby M, case, enforced, where initially courts found indication of a state's intention to prohibit surrogacy arrangements in the fact that they were not expressly authorized[24] and, more latterly, where they have been most accommodating.[25]

Legislative responses have also not been uniform. The UK became, in 1985, the first country to legislate when it passed an ill-considered and largely irrelevant panic measure,[26] which in essence, criminalized commercial surrogacy. The Act was conceived in extravagant terms by some of those who favoured it. Thus, it would 'preserve family life, stabilise society and do away with this unnatural and unfortunate practice which has sickened so many decent-living and family-loving people'[27] and would 'rightly' outlaw 'the hell and wickedness that exists in America – where women are exploited and handled in an undignified manner for gain'.[28] Another Bill to strengthen the law has since failed,[29] but further legislation has been promised.[30] In the USA, before 'Baby M' exploded on the national scene, the legislative climate regarding surrogacy was highly in favour of the practice. Four of five Bills that were pending in the middle of 1986 would have legalized the practice, and California's Assembly had approved a highly deregulated approach to surrogacy. However, following on from 'Baby M', Bills in state legislatures vary: there were 64 bills introduced by 26 jurisdictions in the first half of 1987 and these were evenly split amongst those that prohibit surrogacy arrangements, those that allow them, and those (wisely) calling for more investigation of the issues before surrogacy is banned or legalized.[31] There has also been federal activity with a Democratic Congressman from Ohio introducing a bill modelled on the UK Act of 1985 but broader in its scope.[32] In Australia, Victoria has enacted the most 'comprehensively prohibitive'[33] legislation[34]: in Ontario the most permissive has been proposed with a scheme to regulate what would amount to 'surrogate adoption'.[35]

Meanwhile, there has been opposition to surrogacy from commissions of enquiry such as Warnock,[36] and Waller[37] and Demack[38] and there have been swingeing attacks on the concept by Corea,[39] Duelli-Klein,[40] Radin,[41] Dworkin[42] and other feminists.[43] But the feminist response has not been uniform, as the valuable recent essay by Zipper and Sevenhuissen[44] illustrates. Critical, but more balanced, are the views of Alex Capron[45] and Derek Morgan.[46] Not too much academic literature wholeheartedly supports surrogacy (Robertson's attempt to see surrogacy as an incident and positive aspect of procreative liberty is the clearest endorsement),[47] but a considerable amount, including a previous paper of my own[48] and the valuable essay in Singer and Wells's *The Reproduction Revolution*[49] (as well as dissentients in Warnock)[50] adopt the view, now accepted by the Ontario Commission, that the best way to control the damage that surrogacy could potentially cause is through the process of regulation.[51] What, therefore, is wrong with surrogacy?

Warnock and exploitation

Surrogacy tends to be associated with the new biotechnology, although, of course, it requires no medical intervention,[52] let alone biotechnical skill. But of all the recent aspects of the reproduction revolution it is the one which has provoked the most intense passion and anger. It is significant that commissions such as Warnock, Benda[53] and a Dutch committee[54] which have approved *in vitro* fertilization have condemned surrogacy. Why, for example, did Warnock, in recommending a statutory licensing authority – a proposal now accepted in a Government White Paper – [55] stop short of including surrogacy within its remit?

The Warnock recommendations on surrogacy are the weakest part of the report – a report increasingly recognized as incoherent and philosphically muddled.[56] The Committee was firmly wedded to autonomy on artificial insemination, *in vitro* fertilization, and egg and embryo donation, but on surrogacy it adopted a moralistic, paternalistic position. A woman should not be allowed to use her uterus for financial profit and treat it as an incubator for someone else's child. It is, the Report notes, 'the moral and social objections to surrogacy' that 'weighed heavily' with the Committee.[57] It thought that the weight of public opinion was against the practice of surrogacy,[58] but to move from this assumption to a proposal for criminalization (which it did) is to indulge in an overt enforcement of morality, such as we have come to associate with Lord Devlin,[59] a position from which Lady Warnock would wish, it seems, to distance herself.[60]

Rather surprisingly, when the Report comes to consider surrogacy, it first tackles it 'for convenience alone'.[61] In other words, instead of considering whether, if surrogacy could be justified for the infertile, it could also be defended in the case of fertile women who did not want pregnancy to interfere with a career or, simply perhaps did not wish to be pregnant, the committee reversed the process and started with the more dubious and less common (one could add the less meritorious) case. *Sub silentio* a consequentialist argument is being adduced: look what surrogacy might lead to! The Committee, however, did not apply the 'slippery slope' argument to the case against surrogacy.[62] Instead, it states peremptorily that surrogacy for the fertile is 'totally ethically unacceptable'.[63] It neither tells us whose ethics have imposed this judgement nor offers any appreciation at all of why some women might find the use of surrogates convenient. It gives the following reason: 'that people should treat others as a means to their own ends, however desirable the consequences, must always be liable to moral objection.'[64] If this argument had been applied consistently (and note the use of the word 'always'), no embryo experimentation could be allowed unless (presumably) embryos were not 'others',[65] and artificial insemination by donor, egg donation and embryo donation would also have to be rejected. So, of course, would much else in the medical field (bone marrow transplants, kidney donations, blood transfusions) and, indeed, elsewhere.

The Warnock Report is concerned with the 'serious risk of commercial exploitation'.[66] Warnock herself, in her Introduction, tells us that the Inquiry agreed unanimously that they disapproved of the practice. She tells us that this was 'largely because of possible consequences for the child'.[67] In the Report itself, surrogacy is said to be 'potentially damaging' to the child and also 'degrading'.[68] The Committee, however, concluded that, although surrogacy as a practice was wrong, it could not be prevented by law 'because of the intrusiveness of any law that would be enforceable'.[69] That is why the focus is on 'how surrogacy for commercial purposes might be checked.'[70] The reason for recommending the criminalization of commercial surrogacy is expressed thus:

> Not only was the wrongness of surrogacy compounded by its being exploited for money, but also a law against agencies would not be intrusive into the private lives of those who were actually engaged in setting up a family.[71]

Encapsulated within these paragraphs are the essential objections to surrogacy, found not just in the Warnock Report, but elsewhere in the critical literature. There are any number of secondary attacks on the institution (which are discussed below). Here I will concentrate on the force of the objection that surrogacy is exploitative.

The argument must be carefully stated. The Warnock Report cannot be held to aver that surrogacy is exploitative because the surrogate's body is used to produce a commodity for exchange (a means to an end). For, if this were the argument, then it would have to be conceded, as Marxists indeed claim,[72] that everyday life involves exploitation at every turn. If we accept the Marxist claim, surrogacy becomes yet another example of exploitation in the labour market, but presumably one that is no worse than others. Why, then, condemn it as impermissible, and leave the rest of the social fabric intact? Or is there something very different about using another woman's brains (a teacher or physiotherapist) or a man's brawn (to remove waste from dustbins)? Is the uterus something special? Does a taboo attach to it? Is there a connection between human dignity and sexuality? Is it the association with sexuality that is leading critics to condemn surrogacy?[73]

If this is the Warnock Committee's claim, it is untenable and incongruent. Why single out surrogacy for condemnation? But properly read, the Warnock Report may be held to be asserting that surrogacy exploits because it involves a transaction in which one party is, as a result of circumstances (such as poverty, unemployment), subjected to the demands of another more powerful party. Exploitation in these terms takes place when one person is coerced into doing something she would otherwise not do because she has less power than the exploiter, and when the exploiter uses his advantage of power to force (convince, persuade, coax) her to do as he wishes. The exploiter, in other words, treats the exploited as a means to his end and thus fails to respect her as a person. She is not the subject of 'equal concern and respect'[74] and her autonomy[75] is accordingly thwarted. If this is the Warnock indictment (and it must be made clear again that it is not thus spelt out), surrogacy is being condemned because the surrogate's basic rights to liberty and equality are being undermined. If this is true, it is indeed a powerful indictment of what is assumed to be the typical surrogacy arrangement.

The context of surrogacy: the surrogate's motivation

Before this is examined critically, two points must be made. First, we do not know enough about surrogacy to know what the motivation in the 'typical' case is. Kim Cotton would certainly not consider that she was exploited.[76] Nor would Kirsty Stevens[77] or Mary Stewart.[78] On the other hand Mary-Beth Whitehead would certainly think she got a 'raw deal'[79] and so would the Derbyshire woman at the centre of the case reported in 1987 as Re P[80] (although the court upheld her claim to retain the twins). We can draw no conclusions from the pathological cases that, for one reason or other, are litigated. It is impossible to tell how representative the facts which emerge in these cases are of the norm. How many surrogacy arrangements are altruistic in motivation, even if money changes hands?[81] It is one of the faults of the Warnock Inquiry that, in ignoring the psychological dimensions of surrogacy, it failed to get to grips with what may be a quite common situation, where one woman decides she wishes to help out another less fortunate than herself.

Second, it has to be conceded that many surrogates are indeed poor women. Again, data is patchy, but evidence from the USA does suggest that 40 per cent of surrogacy applicants (in a particular, well publicized sample) were unemployed or on welfare.[82] It would be interesting to know what percentage of a matched sample of applicants for a factory job came into a similar category. I suspect the figure would be similar. The brutal and inescapable fact is that women constitute the 'new poor'. Diana Pearce has referred to this as the 'feminization of poverty'.[83] The poor woman who uses her reproductive abilities to produce a child for an infertile woman and in so doing improves her own standard of living may well not think she is being exploited. Those who see exploitation as inherent in surrogacy may see in this 'false consciousness'.[84] There is some truth in this but it is also patronizing and deflects attention from capitalism generally. The Conservative MPs[85] who saw surrogacy as the unacceptable face of capitalism chose to ignore (or failed to understand) how integral exploitation is to capitalism. They saw exploitation as the pathological side of capitalism and not as part of it.

Surrogacy: liberty and equality

But we must return to the argument that surrogacy is morally wrong because it violates rights to liberty and equality. Does surrogacy necessarily entail the infringement of these basic rights? If an argument could be put that it did there might be a case for banning it, for refusing to allow women to forfeit fundamental rights. But are the rights to liberty and equality damaged irreparably by the activities involved in surrogacy? Is agreeing to become a surrogate akin to selling oneself into slavery? It will be remembered that John Stuart Mill, that high apostle of state non-intervention into the private realm, drew the line, *inter alia*, at selling oneself into slavery.[86] There are those who analogize surrogacy with slavery, as they do with other 'evils'. As a piece of rhetoric or vituperation[87] this is fine, but it does not stand up to analysis. It is worth examining briefly Mill's objection to slavery: it was that the selling of oneself into slavery was an exercise in autonomy which thereafter precluded further exercises in autonomy. But surrogacy involves not the selling of one's body, but of services, and places on those services a very clear time-limit. There are restrictions, it is true, on the way the surrogate may use her body (for example, abstaining from sexual intercourse with her husband during the period surrounding insemination, and not undergoing an abortion) but these cannot be seen as comparable to the incidents of slavery. The use of legal techniques like specific enforcement[88] (countenanced in the Ontario report)[89] do impose slave-like restrictions, but in themselves do not turn that institution into slavery. They will only be invoked at the 'tug-of-love' stage and then a 'best interests of the child' principle is more satisfactory than reliance on contract law.[90]

Surrogacy is not like slavery. But is it, nevertheless, intrinsically exploitative? Cannot a woman freely decide to offer services? Cannot a woman be motivated by the desire to make another couple happy? Why is the concerned, sympathetic, altruistic woman to be labelled as exploited? The fact that she earns money for this service does not mean that she is exploited. Some prostitutes are exploited (by pimps, I suspect, rather than clients) and some exploit their clients, but as many offer a service, and the fact that they are paid for this service does not mean that the relationship thereby becomes one of exploitation.[91] Male–female sexual relations are unequal economic bargains: why then should surrogates or prostitutes be singled out for 'punishment' for something that is pervasive in woman's condition?

At this point it is worth asking what is entailed in the right to liberty. Central to that right, I would argue, is the right to do with your body as you please. On this analysis, the surrogate mother has a right to use her body to give birth to the baby of another. To deny her the decision to become a surrogate thus violates her right to liberty. We can take away liberty-rights. Very few of them are totally unqualified. But the onus rests on those who wish to restrict liberty to put forward sound moral arguments to support limitations on freedom.[92] What arguments can they adduce? The arguments are phrased in various ways (motherhood or woman is dehumanized, children are commodified).[93] The latter argument must be, and is later, addressed in this chapter. But as arguments proferred to buttress limitations on autonomy, they amount to little more than the enforcement of morality for morality's sake (upholding the institution of 'the family',[94] whatever that might mean, to stabilize that equally vague fetish 'society'). And, as such, I do not think the arguments satisfy, for all the reasons used to attack Devlin[95] which need not be rehearsed here.

It might, however, be said that another of the rights to liberty which a surrogate should enjoy is the right to keep the child which (in a partial[96] surrogacy) is genetically half hers and which, whether the surrogacy is partial or total, she may feel psychologically to be hers. This is a forceful argument, but most surrogates do not wish to keep and rear the child they have produced (to order, so to speak). The problem arises in those very few cases where she changes her mind. She will, of course, have waived her right to retain the child.[97] Can she retract her waiver? If the law holds she cannot (as the Superior Court of New Jersey appeared to do in *Baby M*[98]), is it infringing one of her rights to liberty? Is her promise any less binding[99] because of its subject-matter? If she had not entered into the contract freely, there is no reason why she should not retract her waiver. But how widely are we to extend the concept of duress or coercion? Can it really extend to inequality of bargaining power? And what of the surrogate who exploits the commissioning parents by extorting additional sums or promises out of them by threatening to retain the child? These are difficult questions to answer. Fortunately, they only need to be answered in a small minority of cases. And, in those, it is the needs of the 'children of Armageddon'[100] to which our attention should turn, and not questions of rights. At the stage of a dispute, if the surrogate has a right to retain the child (which, given the binding nature of her promise, I think dubious) two rights are in conflict, and a decision is best made on a 'best interests' of the child test, as would be the case in any other custody dispute.[101]

And the child?

What of the child? Warnock, it will be remembered, thought a surrogacy agreement was 'degrading to the child who is to be the outcome of it since . . . the child will have been bought for money'.[102] This is surely fallacious. The money is paid to the surrogate not to compensate her for giving up the child, nor to 'buy' the child. The money is payment for services; it is compensation for the burden of pregnancy. The child may well have a right not to be sold, but that is a distortion of what is happening, even in cases of commercial surrogacy. Does the child have a right to be brought up by his natural parents? This would be difficult in the case of most surrogate births but, even were it not, it is difficult to see how such a right could be constructed[103] or what it would be worth. The child certainly has a right to care and nurture but not, it should be stressed, fom a woman who has agreed to hand him over to others who are intent on offering him or her precisely that.

Thus fleshed out (and using rights arguments only implicit in the Warnock Report), the Warnock case against surrogacy is thin, distorted and unconvincing.

In the course of this discussion some passing reference has been made to other arguments against the practice of surrogacy. These will now be considered at greater length.

Other objections to surrogacy

There are any number of additional possible objections to the practice of surrogacy. Some of these have considerably more force than others, but none, I believe, can ultimately prevail over the common-sense solution of getting to grips with a phenomenon which is here to stay and which, accordingly, I believe should be carefully regulated. It is not an ideal solution, but then it is not an ideal world.

Things go wrong

Some of the objections can be readily disposed of. Thus, it is frequently said that in surrogacy arrangements things often go wrong or just sometimes come to grief. The Stiver–Mallahoff case is a frequently quoted[104] instance. In January 1983 Judy Stiver, a surrogate, delivered a baby with a small head, probably indicating that the child was mentally retarded. All parties involved (the Stivers and the commissioning parents) initially rejected the baby and announced that it would be put up for adoption. The 'father' instructed the hospital to 'take no steps or measures to treat the strep infection or otherwise care for the child'. The hospital successfully applied for an order to allow it to treat the child. On a US TV programme[105] it was alleged that Mallahoff 'asked the hospital to put this baby to sleep, and then he asked [Judy Stiver] to start over and make a new one for him. It's just like buying a defective piece of merchandise'. This was denied by Mallahoff, who contended that he was not the child's father. Blood tests proved him right, and the Stivers agreed to keep the baby. Whatever the ending (and it does have the making of an adult fairytale!), the facts of the Stiver–Mallahoff dispute are undoubtedly sordid. But what conclusions can be drawn from it? Some children are born handicapped and some children are rejected but this also happens in 'normal' families. It has to be conceded that the commissioning parents are more likely to reject a handicapped child. They want a 'normal' child: they could have adopted a handicapped one. The wife may well lack maternal feelings, the commissioning father may feel cheated. There is, I think, no suggestion that the children of surrogates are more likely to be born handicapped. We do not know how common is the incidence of handicap or rejection. To draw conclusions adverse to surrogacy from the Stiver–Mallahoff saga is to indulge in the old maxim that 'hard cases make bad law'. That the Stiver–Mallahoff litigation occurred is unfortunate, but it would be wrong to draw too many conclusions from it.

Disgenic dangers

The objection here is straightforward and clear. The practice of surrogacy could narrow the genetic pool, the result of which would be that the procedure became disgenic. The asssumption behind this fear is that women will become surrogates on multiple occasions. The disgenic danger is lower than in the case of artificial insemination by donor (a man could theoretically make thousands of semen donations) or egg-harvesting, but it is a danger nonetheless. However, it is unlikely that any woman would want to become a surrogate on more than a few occasions or that she would be allowed to do so. One clear advantage of regulation would be to impose limitations and thus to obviate real disgenic dangers. AID is controlled in this way:[106] there is no reason why surrogacy should not be.

Slippery slopes

Surrogacy, Alex Capron said at a Colloquium in Cambridge in September 1987, 'may play the role of entering wedge for more radical changes later'.[107] Put simply, an objection to surrogacy is that if we allow the practice now it will lead to other practices which are inherently undesirable. Williams[108] distinguishes two types of 'slippery slope' argument: the 'horrible result' argument and the 'arbitrary result' argument. Opponents of surrogacy use the 'horrible result' argument (look what is at the bottom of the slope). To an extent this was more than implicit in the Warnock Report, raising the spectre of surrogacy 'for convenience' as an argument against surrogacy even for the infertile.[109] And it is very clearly the fear of some feminists who see a danger that a woman's attributes (her colour, height, intelligence, 'looks') may be 'monetized',[110] that the market value attracted by potential surrogates will vary according to whether they have what are deemed desirable attributes or not. They fear men bypassing their wives (or partners) and using surrogates (tested for the 'right' qualities) to produce their children. They see men, thus enabled, acquiring property interests in their genetic products. This would have far-reaching implications in such areas as abortion,[111] custody and access questions and adoption.[112] And, if a regulating framework is constructed, they envisage this as a further step in the direction of state licensing of pregnancy, with governments prescribing when, how, by whom and in what circumstances women may seek to have children.

None of this, it has to be argued, is a pleasant scenario. Some of it, biotechnology, or not, is already happening, as disputes over contraception,[113] abortion,[114] sterilization,[115] and cases involving the removal of babies at birth[116] amply illustrate. But the real question is: how likely is it that the acceptance of surrogacy will lead to these 'horrible' results? As Williams notes: one can only appeal to such a process when it is 'probable in actual social fact that such a process will occur'. This 'requires that there should be some motive for people to move from one step to the next'. He adds that conservatives sometimes 'simply assume this'.[117] Slippery slope arguments look to both the logical and empirical consequences of the adoption of different policies.[118] But, in this context, it addresses pre-eminently empirical consequences. The problem with the empirical slippery slope argument is that 'it can be used against any proposal that it is capable of misuse'.[119] Thus, for example, those[120] who attacked the decision by the House of Lords to sanction involuntary sterilization of a mentally handicapped girl[121] could point to widespread examples of misuse, in the USA,[122] in Nazi Germany, India and elsewhere. They could also cite the way sterilization had been routinized in this country before an educational psychologist 'blew the whistle'[123] in the 'Sotos Syndrome' case in 1975.[124] But they cannot be certain. They are making evaluations and predictions. And so it is here. Critics of surrogacy can point to all sorts of horrible results, but they cannot say these will happen. Indeed, in comparison with, for example, sterilization, there are no precedents. Some of the results to which they point may, indeed, happen. For example, take Corea's fear that when total surrogacy is actualized, and the surrogate will contribute nothing but a nine-month lease of her womb, Third World women will be used as surrogates and paid a pittance.[125] But surely the point is to stop this happening not by putting a blanket ban on surrogacy, but by sensibly regulating it and thus avoiding the occurrence of this evil. Surrogacy agencies which operated like adoption agencies would not allow this to happen. Of course, a few cases would slip through the net, as they do with adoption.[126] It may, in such cases, be necessary to allow the commissioning parents to adopt despite the iniquity which has occurred: the child's 'best interests' might dictate such a conclusion. But the attack would then focus not on regulated surrogacy but on the exploitation of the unregulated surrogacy arrangement. Adoption as a practice also transfers babies (and children) from the poor to the better off.[127] The fact that it is sometimes practised wrongly does not lead us to condemn the institution outright.[128]

Surrogacy does have dangers, but they are not inevitable consequences of the practice and they can be guarded against.

The commodification of the child

The most substantial argument against surrogacy is that it will have a detrimental effect on children. For too long children have been seen as property rather than persons; they have been reified as social problems, denied participation in decision-making processes about themselves. As a result, children have suffered from many wrongs, including physical violence and sexual abuse. The children's rights movement is trying to redefine childhood and the place the child should occupy in society.[129] A cultural revolution is required, but some progress is being made. Is the development of surrogacy a setback to this progress?

A consequence (or at least a potential consequence) of the emergence of surrogacy is that children may come to be seen as commodities. Look at two models of surrogacy. The first (the purest altruism) may occur when a fertile sister 'gives' her infertile one a child, the product of her ovum and the infertile sister's husband's semen. Note the language: we are talking of 'gifts' and 'products'. In the second model (a commercial surrogacy) the child can clearly be seen as the product of an expensive business transaction. Technically, the commissioning parents may be buying gestational services: they feel they are buying a baby.[130] Furthermore, they want to feel it is at least half 'genetically' theirs. That that half is the man's may itself cause problems.

It was Mia Kellmer-Pringle who attacked the attitude that children complete a family like any other consumer durable (she exampled the TV or fridge).[131] Is surrogacy not encouraging this attitude? You go to a shop to purchase your video and the local surrogacy agency to purchase your child. Just as videos must be of merchantable quality, so too must the child. Fortunately, most children (like most videos) are, so that litigation like the Stiver–Mallahoff case, already referred to, is rare and likely to remain so.

The dangers in turning the baby into a market commodity are graphically portrayed by Radin.

> If a capitalist baby industry were to come into being, with all of its accompanying paraphernalia, how could any of us, even those who did not produce infants for sale, avoid subconsciously measuring the dollar value of our children? How could our children avoid being

preoccupied with measuring their own dollar value? This makes our discourse about ourselves (when we are children) and about our children (when we are parents) like our discourse about cars. In the worst case, market rhetoric could create a commodified self-conception in everyone, as the result of commodifying every attribute that differentiates us and that other people value in us, and could destroy personhood as we know it.[132]

Though exaggerated, I concede that this is a potential danger. However, it is an argument which has something of the 'slippery slope' about it. And in response one must ask: but how likely is it that surrogacy could lead to this? Second, it is premised on the basis of the emergence of a 'capitalist baby industry'. If surrogacy were to be taken over by institutions like adoption agencies, would this happen? It may still be said that adoption agencies deal in existing children (again note the word 'deal') and that surrogacy agencies would be involved in producing children. Like it or not, I think it has to be accepted that, to some extent (which is difficult to measure), children are commodified by the surrogacy transaction, however conducted. There cannot be any doubt that surrogacy poses a threat to our notion of childhood, certainly to an ideal of children for which the children's rights movement strives.

Harm to children

More generally, it may be possible to identify specific harms to which the surrogate child is exposed. There are problems of identity. Who is his or her 'real' mother?[133] The problem is one shared by adopted children, and can be successfully overcome in that context. Social policy encourages an adopted child to know who he or she is and since 1975 (in England, and much earlier in Scotland) an adopted child has had access to his or her original birth certificate.[134] It would be idle to pretend there are no problems. This particular difficulty cannot, however, be said to be major, provided those that need help get it. Post-surrogacy casework may become yet another task of social work in years to come.

The surrogate child may encounter other psychological problems. Why was he or she bought and sold? If this could happen once, why not again? This could clearly pose a threat to the child's sense of security. There may also be burdens on the surrogate child to do well. He or she is an 'investment' and must live up to parents' expectations. These are all problems: it cannot be pretended that we are dealing with a 'normal' parent–child relationship. But I cannot believe they are insuperable. We have enough experience of dealing with children brought up in 'unnatural' environments to be able to provide the sort of assistance and counselling that should enable all but the grossest of problems to be surmounted.

The problem of the surrogate's other children must also be considered. Since most surrogates are likely to be married women with children, these children will observe their mothers carrying babies to term and returning from the maternity hospital empty-handed. If their mother can give the new baby away, then why not them? But this problem can surely be overcome by parents preparing children in advance. And children can be remarkably resilient. Krimmel[135] quotes one 9-year-old girl who, when told that the child her mother was carrying would be given away to another family, responded: 'All right . . . but if it's a girl, let's keep it and give Jeffrey away.' Jeffrey was her 2-year-old brother.

Miscellaneous objections

Six objections to surrogacy have been considered. Only one has been found to be justified: the danger that the practice will commodify children and in doing so obstruct the recognition of the full personality of children. This is a serious charge and cannot be overlooked. For the rest, the objections have been found to be either not proven, speculative or preventable.

But the objections raised are far from the only ones to be found in the literature, although many of the remainder are variants of those already considered. Thus, some would object to surrogacy because it undermines the traditional institution of marriage,[136] though others might respond that assisted procreation may help to stabilize marriage. To others, surrogacy advantages men[137] or the rich[138] (there is said to be a wealth-based access to technology)[139] or leads to a sub-class of underprivileged women (or does it assist some underprivileged women to improve their status? – [140] there is something of a double bind here).

Conclusion

So, what is one to do? In a previous article[141] I argued the case for regulation and, in this chapter, I have indicated how I believe regulation could overcome some of the problems incumbent on surrogacy arrangements. What remains clear to me is that there is a clear demand for surrogacy which will not go away because feminists and others do not like it or because governments ban it. This chapter has demonstrated that the principal objection to surrogacy – that it exploits or dehumanises women – does not stand up to critical examination. The subsidiary argument, that it commodifies children, has more force, particularly in a world in which genuine attempts are being made to improve the child's status. There is a danger that regulating surrogacy will promote it, and, for the reason just given, surrogacy is not to be encouraged. But driving it underground, or to countries which accept it (and international agreement seems most unlikely) will not tackle the problems. If there is exploitation of women, it will be maximized: the evil of baby-selling, and thus the commodification of children, will be aggravated. Regulation can, at least, eliminate the most undesirable elements of the surrogacy practice and, for this reason, I still believe it is preferable to total prohibition or reliance on the instrument of contract.

As I write women march against a Bill[142] which will limit abortion. They do so in the name of a woman's right to use her body as she wishes. Is it not ironic that the main onslaught on surrogacy comes from the very same lobby?

Notes

1   The earliest reported example is the case of *A* v. *C* (1978) 8 Fam. Law 170 (fully reported only in 1985: see [1985] FLR, 445). I am ignoring the oft-cited Biblical examples, which were not true surrogacies.

2   As to which see Cohen, S., *Folk Devils and Moral Panics*, MacGibbon and Kee, 1972; and on surrogacy specifically Dyer, C.; 'Baby Cotton and the Birth of a Moral Panic', the *Guardian* , 15 January 1985 and Hutchinson, A. and Morgan, D., 'A Bill Born from Panic', the *Guardian*, 12 July 1985.

3   Surrogacy Arrangements Act 1985 see commentary by Freeman M. D. A. in *Current Law Statutes Annotated*, London, Sweet & Maxwell, 1986. See also Morgan, **49** *MLR* 1986, 358.

4   In the UK, Warnock (1984); in Canada, the Ontario Law Reform Commission, *Report on Human Artificial Reproduction and Related Matters*, 1985; in Germany, the Benda Commission.

5   The Surrogacy Arrangements Act 1985 (UK); the Infertility (Medical Procedures) Act 1984 (Victoria).

6   See Morgan, D., **12** *JLS*, 1985, 219; Krause **19** *FLQ* 1985, 185; Parker, D. 1984, **14** *Family Law*, 140; Robertson, J. **59**, *South California Law Review*, 1986, 501; Radin, M. 1987, **100** *Harvard Law Review* 1849; Capron A., 1987, **20** *U.C. Davis Law Review* 679; Stumpf, A. R. **96** *Yale Law Journal* 1986, 187. Also most valuable is Easlea, B., *Science and Sexual Oppression*, London, Weidenfeld and Nicolson, 1981.

7   Corea, G., *The Mother Machine*, Harper and Row, 1985 (ch. 11 is the best). See also Corea, G. *et al. Man-Made Women*, London, Hutchinson, 1985; Dworkin, A., *Right-Wing Women*, New York, Perigee Books, 1983; Overall, C. (1986) **1** *CJWI*, 271; see also Radin M., *op. cit.*, note 6. Ironically, Shulamith Firestone, *The Dialect of Sex*, New York, Murrow, 1970 saw the new birth technology as liberating for women.

8   Estimates vary. The Ontario Law Reform Commission, *Report*, op. cit., (note 4) vol. 1, p. 10 makes this estimate.

9   According to Knoppers, B. M., *Family Law in Canada: New Directions*, Canadian

Advisory Council on the Status of Women, 1985, p. 214, it has increased in Canada by 83 per cent between 1965 and 1979. The increase may be attributed to the practice of abortion and contraceptive techniques, in particular the 'coil'. More resources are put into biotechnology than in reducing risks to fertility – a common criticism in feminist writing.

10   See Bromley, P., 'Aided conception: the alternative to adoption' in Bean, P. (ed.), *Adoption: Essays in Social Policy, Law and Sociology*, London, Tavistock, 1984, pp. 174–93.

11   See Harriett Blankfield of National Center for Surrogate Parenting in Chevy Chase, Maryland, USA, quoted in Corea, G., *The Mother Machine*, op. cit., note 7, p. 218: 'When it came to wanting a child . . . they didn't want to take what they would consider second-best.' Even if 'they' did, this ignores the difficulties surrounding adoption, particularly of children from the 'Third World'.

12   As to which see Mary Ann Glendon, *Abortion and Divorce in Western Law*, Harvard University Press 1987 (Austria, Denmark, Greece, Norway, Sweden and the USA are characterized as permitting abortion on demand at pp. 151–4). British law was liberalized in 1967 (Abortion Act 1967). There have been countless attempts to restrict access to abortion since. As I write, a Bill to do just this is before Parliament and is reckoned to stand a chance of being successful.

13   In particular for young women who earlier would have provided the 'first-class' babies for adoption. And see now also the landmark decision of *Gillick* v. *West Norfolk and Wisbech AHA* [1986] AC 112.

14   The subtitle of Singer P. and Wells, D., *The Reproduction Revolution*, Oxford University Press, 1984 (still the best introduction to the subject).

15   See Hall, R. V., *A Spy's Revenge*, Harmondsworth, Penguin, 1987.

16   *Baby M*, (1987) 13 Fam. L. Rep. (US) 22, 2001.

17   (1985) FLR 846 or, more personally, Cotton, K. and Winn, D., *Baby Cotton: For Love or Money*, London, Dorling Kindersley, 1985.

18   *Infertility in Women: Diagnosis and Treatment*, Philadelphia, F. A. Davis, 1966, p. 178.

19   Which, if implemented, would give us the 'pre-conception adoption'. See op. cit., note 4, Ontario Law Reform Commission.

20   *A* v. *C* [1985] FLR 445.

21   (1985) FLR 846.

22   *Re Adoption Application* 212/86, *The Times*, 12 March 1986. The surrogate tells her story in Stevens, K., *Surrogate Mother: One Woman's Story*, London, Century, 1985.

23   *Syrkowski* v. *Appleyard* (1985) 362 NW 2d 211; *Doe* v. *Kelley* (1981) 307 NW 2d 438.

24   *Kentucky ex rel. Armstrong* v. *Surrogate Parenting Assoc. Inc.* (1985) 11 Fam. L. Rep. 1359, reversed in *Surrogate Parenting Associates, Kentucky ex. rel. Armstrong* (1986) 704 SW 2d 209.

25   *John Smith and Mary Smith* v. *Mike Jones and Jane Jones* (a decision of the Detroit Wayne County Circuit in 1986).

26   See Freeman, M. D. A., **39** *CLP*, 33 1986, pp. 37–48. One way round the Act has been to pay surrogates to keep a pregnancy diary 'for research purposes'. See *Daily Telegraph*, 15 May 1986.

27   *Hansard*: HC vol. 77, col. 43 *per* Peter Bruinvels MP.

28   *Hansard*: HC vol. 77, col. 45 *per* Harry Greenaway MP.

29   Surrogacy Arrangements (Amendment) Bill 1986, sponsored by the Earl of Halsbury.

30   In the DHSS White Paper *Human Fertilisation and Embryology: A Framework for Legislation* Cm. 259, November 1987.
31   13 FLR 1442 (1987). The Bills which got furthest are those in Arkansas which allowed surrogacy contracts, and which were passed by the legislature, but vetoed by the Governor, and a Bill in Louisiana which provides that contracts for surrogate motherhood 'shall be absolutely null and void and unenforceable as contrary to public policy'. This awaits the Governor's approval at the time of writing.
32   HR 2243. This would amend 18 USC 80 to prohibit making, engaging in or brokering a surrogacy arrangement on a 'commercial basis'. It would also amend 15 USC 52 to prohibit the advertising of the availability of such a commercial surrogacy arrangement.
33   *Per* Dickens B., Legal aspects of surrogate motherhood: practices and proposals', Paper to UK National Committee of Comparative Law 1987 Colloquium, Cambridge, p. 21.
34   Infertility (Medical Procedures) Act 1984 (not yet operative).
35   *Per* Ontario Law Reform Commission, *Report*, op. cit., vol. II, pp. 218–72.
36   The Warnock Report, Cmnd. 9314, 1984, republished (with additional material) as Warnock, M., *A Question of Life*, Oxford, Blackwell, 1985.
37   Waller, L., *Report on the Disposition of Embryos Produced by In Vitro Fertilisation*, 1984, para. 4.17 ('Surrogacy arrangements [should] in no circumstances be made at present as part of an IVF programme in Victoria).
38   *Special Committee Appointed by the Queensland Government to Enquire into the Law relating to Artificial Insemination, In Vitro Fertilisation and other related Matters*, 1984.
39   Corea, G., *The Mother Machine*, New York, Harper & Row, 1985, ch. 11; see also her *Man-Made Women*, Hutchinson, 1985.
40   See Duelli-Klein, R., 'What's new about the "new" reproductive technologies' in Corea, *Man-Made Women*, op. cit., note 39, pp. 64–73.
41   Radin, M., Market-Inalienability', **100** *Harvard Law Review*, 1987, no. 1849, pp. 1928–.
42   Dworkin, A., *Right-Wing Women*, London, Perigee Books, 1983.
43   See Arditti R., *et al. Test-Tube Women*, London Pandora Press, 1984.
44   Zipper, J. and Sevenhuijsen, S., 'Surrogacy: feminist notions of motherhood reconsidered' in Stanworth, *Reproductive Techniques*, Cambridge, Polity Press, 1987, p. 118.
45   Capron, A., **20** *UC Davis Law Review*, 1987, 679. See also 'AID, embryo research and surrogate motherhood: public policy and the constitution', Paper to UK National Committee of Comparative Law Colloquium, 1987.
46   Morgan, D., 'Making motherhood male' **12** *Journal of the Law Society*, 1985, 219; 'Technology and the political economy of reproduction', in Freeman, M. D. A. (ed.), *Medicine, Ethics and the Law*, London, Sweet & Maxwell, 1988.
47   Robertson, J., **595** *Californian Law Review*, 1986, 501. See also 'Procreative liberty, embryos and collaborative reproduction', Paper to UK National Committee of Comparative Law Colloquium, 1987.
48   Freeman, M. D. A., 'After Warnock – whither the law?' (1986) **39** *CLR*, 33.
49   Singer, P., and Wells, D., *The Reproduction Revolution*, Oxford University Press, 1984, ch. 4.
50   Wendy Greengross and David Davies. See also Davies, D., 'Hire-a-womb with safeguards', *The Times*, 19 July 1984 and cf. Warnock, 'Legal surrogacy – not for love or money?', *The Listener*, 24 January 1985.
51   Law Reform Commission Report on *Human Artificial Reproduction and Related Matters*, 1985. There is a powerful dissent by the Vice-Chairman.
52   Total surrogacy, which is dependent on *in vitro* fertilization, of course, does.

There has been (so far as is known) no total surrogacy within Britain yet, though *The Observer* 9 March 1986 reported that plans were afoot at Bourne Hall to use *in vitro* fertilization techniques to accomplish total surrogacy births.

53 Benda, *In-Vitro Fertilisation, Genomanylse und Gentherapie*, Bonn, 1985.
54 *Interimadvies Inzake In Vitro Fertilsatie*, Den Hang, 1984, Gezondheidsraad.
55 Op. cit., note 30.
56 See, for example, Lee, S., 'Re-reading Warnock' in Byrne, P. (ed.), *Rights and Wrongs in Medicine*, King Edward's Hospital Fund for London, 1986, pp. 37–52; Lockwood, M., 'The Warnock Report: a philosophical appraisal' in Lockwood, M. (ed), *Moral Dilemmas In Modern Medicine*, Oxford University Press, 1985, pp. 155–86.
57 Op. cit., note 36, para 8.17.
58 Ibid., para. 8.10. The two dissentients (see note 50) did not believe that public opinion 'is yet fully formed on the question of surrogacy'. This is surely correct if we are talkng of informed public opinion, though there may well be 'widespread intolerance, indignation and disgust' towards the practice (*cf.* Lord Devlin, *The Enforcement of Morals*, Oxford University Press, 1965, p. 17). On public opinion in New South Wales, see New South Wales Law Reform Commission, *Surrogate Motherhood: Australian Public Opinion*, 1987. 51 per cent of respondents were not opposed to surrogate motherhood and 33 per cent did object. The difference in attitude of men and women was marginal.
59 Lord Devlin, *The Enforcement of Morals, op. cit.*, note 58.
60 In the Introduction to *A Question of Life* (op. cit. note 36), Lady Warnock attacks Devlin's consensus view of morality as a 'myth' (p. xi). See also (1986) 39 CLP 17, and 'The artificial family' in Lockwood, M. (ed.) *Moral Dilemmas, op. cit.*, pp. 138–54, at pp. 153–4 particularly.
61 Op. cit., note 36, para. 8.17.
62 On which see Williams, B., 'Which slopes are slippery?' in Lockwood, M. (ed.) *Moral Dilemmas, op. cit.* 126–37.
63 Op. cit., note 36, para. 8.17.
64 *Idem.*
65 A valuable introduction to which is Hursthouse, R., *Beginning Lives*, Oxford, Blackwell, 1987. See also CIBA Foundation, *Human Embryo Research: Yes or No?*, Tavistock, 1986.
66 Op. cit., note 36, para. 8.18.
67 Introduction to Warnock, *A Question of Life, op. cit.*, p. xii.
68 Op. cit., note 36, para. 8.11.
69 Introduction to Warnock, *A Question of Life op. cit.*; p. xii.
70 *Idem.*
71 *Idem.*
72 A good critical treatment of this is Elster, J., *An Introduction to Karl Marx*, Cambridge University Press, 1986, ch. 5. The best treatment is by Roemer, J., *A General Theory of Exploitation and Class*, Harvard University Press, 1982. See also two articles in (1982) **11** *Philosophy and Public Affairs*, 1982, 281–13; **14** *Philosophy and Public Affairs*, 30–65. The question whether workers are coerced to sell their labour power is discussed by Cohen, G. *Philosophy and Public Affairs*, 3–33 and Zimmerman, D., **10** *Philosophy and Public Affairs*, 1981, 121–45.
73 But cf. Andrea Dworkin's comment that 'the only time you hear institutional people . . . discuss women's equality or women's freedom is in the context of equal rights to prostitution, equal rights to some form of selling of the body, selling of the self . . ., something for which there usually *is* no analogy

with men but a specious analogy is being made' (quoted in *The Mother Machine*, op. cit., note 7, pp. 227–8).

74 See Dworkin, R., *Taking Rights Seriously*, London, Duckworth, 1977, pp. 180–3, pp. 272–8.

75 The *locus classicus* of which is Mill, J. S., *On Liberty* (originally published in 1859); see also now Raz, J., *The Morality of Freedom*, Oxford University Press, 1986.

76 She comes across in her story Cotton and Winn, *Baby Cotton*, op. cit., note 15, as a true woman of Finchley, a good entrepreneur (although she has rather more heart than her MP!).

77 See Stevens, *Surrogate Mother*, op. cit.

78 *Social Work Today*, 10 December 1984, p. 14.

79 A reading of that judgement gives clear signs of a class, status and education bias against the surrogate.

80 *Re P* [1987] 2 FLR, 421. She is reported as having said that she wanted the father as well as the twins.

81 According to an article in *The New York Times*, 18 January 1987, whilst potential surrogate mothers stated that their primary motivation was altruism, 89 per cent of those interviewed said 'they would not do it without being paid'.

82 Parker, P., **140** *American Journal of Psychiatry*, 1983, 117. Parker is an associate of Noel Keane, the pioneering surrogacy lawyer. One description of the surrogacy 'industry' at work is Ince, S. 'Inside the surrogate industry' in Arditti, R. *et al.* (eds), *Test-Tube Women*, Pandora Press, 1984, pp. 99–116.

83 Pearce, D., 'The feminization of poverty: women, work and welfare', *Urban and Social Change Review*, 1978.

84 On which, particularly in relation to autonomy, see Lindley, R., *Autonomy*, London, Macmillan, 1987, ch. 10.

85 For example, David Amess M.P., *Hansard*: HC vol. 55, col. 46.

86 Mill, J. S., *On Liberty* (Penguin Edition by G. Himmelfarb), 1974, p. 173.

87 *Per* Dickens B., op. cit., note 33, *supra*, p. 14.

88 See Singer, P. and Wells, D., *The Reproduction Revolution*, Oxford University Press, 1984, pp. 121–3. The problem is also discussed in Keane, N. and Breo, D, *The Surrogate Mother* New York, Everest House 1981.

89 Op. cit., note 4, *supra*.

90 As in *Re P* [1987] 2 FLR 421. Cf. the approach in *Baby M*, op. cit.

91 When surrogacy is compared with prostitution, the implicit assumption seems to be that prostitution is wrong, but the justification for this judgment is never spelt out. Cf. Richards, D., *Sex, Drugs, Death and the Law*, New Jersey, Roman and Littlefield, 1982, pp. 84–127 (Kantian autonomy permits commercial sex) and Ericsson, L., **90**, *Ethics*, 1980, 335, with Pateman, C., **93** *Ethics* 1983, 561. See also Radin op. cit., note 6 supra, pp. 1921–5.

92 See Hart, H. L. A., *Law, Liberty and Morality*, Oxford University Press, 1963.

93 See the arguments of Radin, op. cit., note 6, pp. 1855–9, 1925–36.

94 See David, M., 'Moral and maternal: the family in the right' in Levitas, R. (ed.) *The Ideology of the New Right*, 1986 and Lewis, J. and Cannell, F., 'The politics of motherhood in the 1980s', **13** *JLS* 1986, 321–42. Also useful is Mellows, D. **8** *Harvard Women's Law Journal*, 1985, 23.

95 For instance in Hart, *Law, Liberty and Morality*, supra cit., note 92, or Dworkin, R., *Taking Rights Seriously*, Duckworth, 1977, ch. 10.

96 That is one produced by artificial insemination or by natural intercourse with the father, as opposed to *in vitro* fertilization using the ovum of another woman.

97 This is a standard term in the contracts found in the USA.

98 *Baby M* (1987) 13 Fam L Rep (US) 22 2001 (discussed by Rachels, J., **1** *Bioethics*,

1987, 357–65. This has been reversed by the Supreme Court of New Jersey (see *New York Times*, 4 February, 1988).

99 On contracts as binding promises see Fried, C., *Contract As Promise*, Harvard University Press, 1981 and Atiyah, P., *Promises, Morals and Law*, Oxford University Press, 1981. See, further, Moor, A., 'Are contracts promises?' in Eekelaar, J. and Bell, J. (eds), *Oxford Essays in Jurisprudence*, (3rd series), Clarendon Press, 1987, pp. 103–24.

100 The phrase (coined by A. Watson: see **21** *Syracuse Law Review*, 1980, p. 55) describes the children caught in the crossfire of divorce.

101 See J. *v.* C [1970] A.C. 668, 710; *S(BD)* v. *S(DJ)* [1977] Fam. 109.

102 Op. cit. note 36, *supra*.

103 On the problems of which see Freeman, M. D. A., *The Rights and Wrongs of Children'*, Pinter, 1983, ch. 2.

104 Discussed in Corea, op. cit., note 7, pp. 219–20, 230 and Singer, P. and Wells D., op. cit., note 88, pp. 118–19.

105 The Donahue show, as quoted in Corea, op. cit, note 7, p. 218.

106 And see the recommendations in the Warnock Report, op. cit., note 36, para 4.26.

107 See Paper to UK National Committee of Comparative Law Colloquium, op. cit., note 45, p. 24.

108 Williams, op. cit., note 62.

109 See para 8.17.

110 *Radin*, op. cit., note 6, *supra* p. 1857.

111 See *Paton* v. *British Pregnancy Advisory Service Trustees* [1979] QB 276; C. v. S [1987] 1 All ER 1230 (the aftermath of this case is described in *The Sunday Times*, 17 January 1988).

112 See *Re C (MA)* [1966] 1 All E.R. 838; *Re TD* [1985] FLR 1150. See also the Family Law Reform Act 1987, particularly s. 4.

113 See *Gillick* v. *West Norfolk and Wisbech* AHA [1986] AC 112.

114 See *C.* v. *S* [1987] 1 All ER 1230 and the debate over the reform of the Abortion laws in 1988.

115 *Re B* [1987] 2 All ER 206; *Re T, The Independent*, 14 July 1987.

116 *D* v. *Berkshire CC.* [1987] 1 All ER 20; *Re F, The Times*, 20 January 1988. See also the *Raynor* saga of November 1987 (for example in *The Times*, 11 November 1987).

117 Williams, op. cit., note 62, p. 132.

118 And see Williams, B., *Ethics and the Limits of Philosophy*, London, Fontana, 1985.

119 Gillon R., 'On sterilising severely mentally handicapped people', **13**, *Journal of Medical Ethics*, 1987, 59, 61.

120 Including myself (see 'Sterilising the mentally handicapped' in Freeman, M. D. A. (ed.), *Medicine, Ethics and the Law*, London, Sweet and Maxwell, 1988.

121 The Jeanette case (see *Re B*, op. cit., note 115).

122 See Meyers, D., *The Human Body and the Law*, Edinburgh University Press, 1971, ch. 2.

123 Becker, M., *Outsiders*, London, New York, Free Press, 1963, p. 122.

124 [1976] Fam. 185.

125 Corea, op. cit., note 7, p. 215.

126 Independent placements for adoption were banned in 1982, but private fostering arrangements leading to adoptions still take place. See, further Baker, N., *Babyselling: The Scandal of Black-Market Adoptions*, New York, Vanguard Press, 1978.

127 See Benet, M. K., *The Character of Adoption*, Jonathan Cape, 1976; Holman, R., 'A class analysis of adoption', *Community Care*, 26 April, 1978, p. 13;

Schorr, A., *Children and Decent People*, London, Allen and Unwin, 1975, p. 188. See also V. MacLeod's statement that implicit in the Children Act 1975 is the view that 'it is either . . . not cost effective to support struggling families, or that substitute families quite frequently provide a better environment for children than natural families' (*Whose Child?*, Study Commission on the Family, 1982, p. 57).

128 Shawyer, J., *Death by Adoption*, New Zealand, Cicada Press, 1979.

129 Freeman, M. D. A., *The Rights and Wrongs of Children*, op. cit.; Franklin, B., *The Rights of Children*, Oxford, Blackwell, 1986.

130 Typically, money changes hands (according to the contract) when the baby is handed over and parental rights are transferred.

131 Kellmer-Pringle, M., *The Needs of Children*, London, Hutchinson, 1977, pp. 69–70.

132 Radin, op. cit., note 6, *supra*, p. 1926.

133 See Triseliotis, J.; *In Search of Origins*, London, RKP, 1973; Triseliotis, J., 'Identity and adoption' **78** *Child Adoption*, 1974, 27–34. Triseliotis, J., 'Identity and security in adoption and long-term forstering', **7**(1) *Adoption and Fostering*, 1983, 22–31; Sorosky, A. D., Baran A., and Panner, R., 'The reuinion of adoptees and birth relatives', **3**(3) *Journal of Youth and Adolescence* 1974, 195–206.

134 Children Act 1975, s. 26 (now Adoption Act 1976 s. 51)

135 Krimmel, H., 'The case against surrogate parenting', Hastings Center Report, October 1983, p. 35.

136 Ibid. Krimmel also makes the point that the legalization of surrogacy arrangements may lead to family breakdown. See also Magisterium of the Catholic Church, *Instruction in Respect for Human Life*, 22 February 1987.

137 'The characterization of the interaction [is] an expression of gender hierarchy. The would-be father is "producing" a baby of his "own" but in order to do so he must purchase these "services" as a necessary input' *per* Radin, op. cit. note 6 *supra*, pp. 1929–30, and see n. 276.

138 A point made by A. Capron.

139 Idem.

140 Zipper and Sevenhuijsen, op. cit., note 44, p. 128.

141 Freeman, M. D. A., 'After Warnock – whither the law?' loc. cit.

142 To amend the Abortion Act 1967. They lost the first round when the Bill got a Second Reading by 45 votes (see *The Independent*, 23 January 1988). The Bill did finally fail, though it is expected to be reintroduced in the next session of Parliament.

8 Reducing maternal mortality: a priority for human rights law

REBECCA COOK

Introduction

It has become easy in the industrialized world to presume that women will normally survive pregnancy. Safe, reliable and legal means of contraception, voluntary sterilization and abortion have significantly reduced pregnancy-related mortality and morbidity. Further, sufficient levels of general health care and advances in prenatal and obstetric care have rendered the overwhelming majority of high-risk pregnancies successfully manageable. Accordingly, we have become complacent about maternal death outside specialized branches of medicine and nursing, and outside what we believe are unrepresentative incidents or anecdotes of our own experience.

Maternal deaths are defined as deaths among women who are pregnant or have been pregnant during the previous 42 days.[1] It is stunning to realize the prevalence of maternal deaths in the world today. Dr Hafdan Mahler, Director General of the World Health Organization (WHO) emphasized in early 1987 that:

> The most striking fact about maternal health in the world today is the extraordinary difference in maternal death rates between industrialised and developing countries. In the industrialised countries maternal deaths are now rare: the average lifetime risk for a woman dying of pregnancy-related causes is between 1 in 4,000 and 1 in 10,000. For a woman in the developing countries the average risk is between 1 in 15 and 1 in 50. These countries commonly have maternal mortality rates 200 times higher than those of Europe and North America – the widest disparity in all statistics of public health.[2]

Less than a century ago the industrialized world experienced similar rates of maternal mortality.[3] Within Western cultures there is an historical sense in which human reproduction can be said to have affected the values of men and the bodies of women.[4] Women's health in itself was not a high priority in the value-system of Western cultures and the laws they created. The duty of women was principally to bear men's children, particularly sons, and to serve as the foundation and the founders of families.[5] The cost of discharging this duty on women's health, and the effects of women's ill health upon their families, went unrecognized. Ill health, influenced perhaps by early and excessive childbearing, and women's premature deaths in labour or from weakness or exhaustion consequent on childbearing, were explained through fate, destiny and divine will. They were not considered amenable to human control through reproductive health programmes and education.

Today, epidemiological and related data show how reproductive health care can reduce both maternal[6] and infant and child mortality,[7] and that health programmes can contribute significantly to the creation and survival of healthy family life.[8] Data also show how the absence of maternal, infant and child health services leave mothers, infants, children and families at risk of sickness and death.[9]

Reproductive safety, both of men and women but particularly of women, raises sensitive issues in the common law tradition because it relates to human sexuality and affects the moral order. The moral belief under the law was that, if humans can indulge in 'easy' sexual relations, without constant liability to pregnancy and the maintenance of children, sexual morality and family security would be in jeopardy. This traditional morality was expressed as recently as 1954 in the celebrated and unduly influential dissenting observation of Lord Justice Denning (as he then was), expressly disapproved by the majority of the English Court of Appeal, regarding vasectomy. He said:

> Take a case where a sterilisation operation is done so as to enable a man to have the pleasure of sexual intercourse without shouldering the responsibilities attached to it. The operation then is plainly injurious to the public interest. It is degrading to the man himself. It is injurious to his wife and to any woman whom he may marry, to say nothing of the way it opens to licentiousness.[10]

Little concession was made to vasectomy inspired by the medical desirability of sparing a wife the hazards of future pregnancy. Lord Denning MR showed the same inclination to favour a vision of the public interest over the health of women in his 1980 decision in *The Royal College of Nursing* case.[11] He considered that Britain's Abortion Act of 1967 did not legally protect later-developed safer techniques of performing abortion which depended on nursing services, finding that, since nurses could not act in terms of the legislation, 'the doctor will have to use the surgical method with its extra hazards'[12] or that the abortion would not be performed. The House of Lords subsequently reversed the Court of Appeal's decision, and upheld the Act's applicability to modern abortion methods, which reduce hazards to women's health.[13]

In many countries, the law presents obstacles to medical and other pursuit of reproductive health.[14] At risk in several areas is not simply health, but life itself. Data are reviewed below of how pregnancy and childbirth are causatively related to deaths of women. Legal accommodation of birth spacing and other family planning practices could prevent many such deaths. The status of common clinic practices, national legislation and case law, which obstruct reproductive choice is reviewed below in the context of international human rights law. The purpose of this chapter is to present the basis of the argument that countries are obligated by international human rights law to reduce maternal mortality. These human rights obligations are addressed by examining rights recognized in legal instruments and by showing how they might be usefully applied to argue for the reduction of maternal mortality.

Maternal mortality

Measurements

The World Health Organization estimates that 500,000 maternal deaths occur annually in the world, about 99 per cent of them in the developing world.[15] Judith Fortney explains that maternal mortality is measured in different ways and the implications will differ depending on which sorts of measurements are used.[16] What is commonly referred to as the maternal mortality rate is actually a ratio of maternal deaths to each 100,000 live births. It is a ratio of maternal deaths to live births and really measures obstetric risk. This measurement of the maternal mortality ratio is likely to be reduced by significant improvement in obstetric care.[17]

Fortney further explains that the actual maternal mortality rate is a true rate and is defined as maternal death per year relative to the number of women aged 15–49:

$$\frac{\text{maternal deaths}}{\text{number of women aged 15–49}} \times 100,000$$

This rate measures both the prevalence of pregnancy and the risk of dying as a result of pregnancy.[18] The rate of maternal mortality is influenced both by better obstetric care which reduces the risk of dying as a result of pregnancy and family planning which reduces the number of pregnancies.[19]

Another way to examine maternal deaths is by reference to the lifetime risk of dying from complications of pregnancy and is variously defined as:

— pregnancy to women of less than 20 years and of more than 39 years and at parity (number of children) of six or more;
– pregnancy to women of less than 18 years of age and more than 35 or 30 and at parity, four or more.[20]

If high-risk pregnancies are reduced, the lifetime risk of dying from complications of pregnancy is reduced. Moreover, if the number of pregnancies is reduced by, for example, better access to means of family planning, the lifetime risk of dying from pregnancy is reduced.[21]

The first of these measurements, the ratio of maternal deaths per 100,000 live births, is the most common and will be used here in discussing the prevalence of maternal death. Maternal mortality ratio tends to differ by region, country, and by area within a country.

In Africa, for instance, maternal mortality ratios range from 166 to 1,100 deaths per 100,000 live births:[22] high maternal mortality ratios are compounded by high fertility – an average of eight live births per woman and hence probably at least 10 pregnancies per woman. An African woman's lifetime risk of dying from pregnancy-related causes is often greater than 1 in 20.[23]

Maternal mortality ratios in Asia vary from 55 deaths in Eastern Asia to 650 deaths per 100,000 live births in Southern Asia.[24] Community studies in rural Anhdra Pradesh, India found a ratio of 874 deaths per 100,000 births.[25] They indicated that 59 per cent of maternal deaths that occur annually occur in Southern Asia.[26]

The extent of maternal death is masked by under-reporting. In Jamaica, for instance, where the official maternal mortality ratio was 48 deaths per 100,000 live births, a national study uncovered an actual ratio of 102 deaths.[27] Hospital data are reliable in themselves, but, of course, exclude maternal deaths outside hospitals. In Nigeria, for example, the hospital maternal mortality ratio was reported in 1985 at 1,050 deaths per 100,000 births.[28]

Causes

The causes of maternal mortality are varied and complex.[29] Dr Mahler explained in his 1987 speech that:

> The cause of a maternal death often has some of its roots in a woman's life before the pregnancy. It may lie in infancy, or even before her birth, when deficiencies of calcium, vitamin D, or iron begin. Continued throughout childhood and adolescence, these faults may result in a contracted pelvis and eventually in death from obstructed labour or in chronic iron-deficiency anaemia and often death from haemorrhage. The train of negative factors goes on through the woman's life; the special risks of adolescent pregnancy; the maternal depletion from pregnancies too closely spaced; the burdens of heavy physical labour in the reproductive period; the renewed high risk of childbearing after 35 and, worse, after 40; the compounding risks of grand multiparity; and running through all this, the ghastly dangers of illegal abortion to which sheer desperation may drive her. All these are like links in a chain from which only the grave or the menopause offer hope of escape.[30]

Thus, there are many factors which can contribute to maternal deaths, and some factors combine with others to compound the risk of death faced by pregnant women.[31] For the purposes of this discussion, obstetric, health service and reproductive factors will be discussed in sequence.

Obstetric factors

Maternal deaths are usually divided into three categories: 'direct' obstetric deaths – those resulting from complications of pregnancy, delivery or their management; 'indirect' obstetric deaths – those due to other medical factors which were aggravated by pregnancy, for example, heart disease or anaemia; and unrelated deaths – fortuitous deaths while pregnant, for example, from accidents.[32]

Most maternal deaths in the developing world are direct obstetric deaths. The major causes of these deaths are haemorrhage, infection and toxaemia (pregnancy-induced hypertension and high blood pressure). Other causes of obstetric death include unskilled abortion, obstructed labour due in part to a deformed pelvis which can arise from chronic malnutrition, and a ruptured uterus.[33] Some of these factors will contribute more than others to maternal mortality. For example, Dr Mahler estimated that 20–50 per cent of the 500,000 maternal deaths occurring annually could be averted by access to safe abortion and contraceptive services.[34] Obviously, in countries where safe abortion is widely available, a programme to reduce maternal mortality will have to analyse other factors carefully.

Health service factors

Health services are deficient in the developing world particularly in the rural areas. Health personnel are inadequately trained and those that are trained are in very short supply. As a result, mistaken or inadequate treatment by health personnel can often be a contributing factor in maternal deaths.[35] Lack of essential supplies such as food and drugs and lack of maternity services or limited access to such services are other contributory factors.

Lack of prenatal care is a significant contributing factor. Prenatal care, whilst not the only answer to reducing maternal mortality among women with high-risk pregnancies, helps to identify such women and increases chances that they are referred to clinics which have appropriately trained health personnel to deal with them.[36] Prenatal care without such back-up referral services is obviously likely to be less effective in reducing maternal mortality from high-risk pregnancies.

Reproductive factors

Deborah Maine and her colleagues explain that family planning can prevent maternal deaths in two ways.[37] The first is by reducing the number of pregnancies. For example, 'If the average number of children per woman is eight (as in Kenya), and use of family planning reduces this number to six, then an average woman's lifetime risk of maternal death is reduced by one-quarter.'[38]

Another way in which family planning prevents maternal deaths, they explain, is by averting high-risk pregnancies.[39] It is well known[40] that the risks of morbidity and mortality associated with pregnancy are greater for women in the following categories:

1   women less than 18 years old;
2   women 35 years and older;
3   women whose last birth occurred in the previous 24 months;
4   women with four or more births;
5   women, such as those who live in a rural area, with limited access to reproductive health services; and
6   women with unwanted pregnancies liable to end in unskilled abortion.

1   *Adolescent pregnancy* Marriage and childbearing at an early age are particularly prevalent both in the developing world and in

low socioeconomic classes in some developed countries. Both are associated with high obstetrical risk and lead to a high incidence of maternal mortality in the adolescent age group. In Botswana, 28 per cent of women who have ever been pregnant are pregnant before reaching the age of 18.[41] In Nigeria, one-quarter of all women are married by the age of 14, one-half by the age of 16 and three-quarters by the age of 18.[42]

Adolescent pregnancies are often associated with high obstetrical risks because adolescents evidently tend not to seek care until late in pregnancy, even when it is easily available.[43] Obstetric factors leading to high prevalence of maternal deaths among adolescents include toxaemia, anaemia and premature labour.[44] In certain situations, adolescents will seek unskilled abortion, such as where they are stigmatized for example by being expelled from school on grounds of their pregnancy.[45] In a study undertaken in Kenyatta National Hospital on mortality due to abortion, 24 per cent of the deaths were among adolescents.[46]

High rates of adolescent pregnancy and high obstetric risks all contribute to high prevalence of maternal mortality in this age group. It has been found that in Jamaica and Nigeria, for instance, women younger than 15 years of age are four to eight times more likely to die during pregnancy and childbirth than women aged 15–19.[47] In the developed world, the maternal death rate for mothers under age 15 has been found to be 2.5 times higher than the rate among mothers aged 20 to 24.[48] It has also been found that in rural Bangladesh, for instance, among women aged 15 to 19, almost 6 in 10 of all deaths are related to pregnancy and childbirth.[49]

2 *Advanced maternal age* Conducted studies have shown high maternal mortality rates for older women. In Bangladesh and Jamaica studies have shown that, when compared to women aged 20–24, those aged 35–39 were between 85–461 per cent more likely to die from a given pregnancy.[50] In England and Wales, women aged 40 or older had at least five times the risk of death in childbirth than did women aged 20–24.[51] Aggravating pregnancy relatively late in reproductive life are high parity (number of births) (see (4) below) and the natural consequences of advancing years. The risk of haemorrhage rises sharply with age, the toxaemias become more frequent amongst older mothers, and the risk of sepsis increases. Ageing disorders, such as cardiovascular disease, make older women especially susceptible to pregnancy complications.

3 *Short birth spacing* This factor directly relates to infant and child mortality[52] and indirectly to maternal mortality. Among women with poor nutrition, pregnancy following soon after childbirth

creates a greater risk of death than is faced by those whose physical status has recovered from earlier childbearing. Infant and child deaths associated with close birth spacing themselves impose health risks on mothers due to higher parity (see (4) below) since family incentives are created to conceive a replacement child.

A mother with a young dependent child may be impaired in obtaining prenatal care during a subsequent pregnancy. The short spacing of births also may be associatedd with the risks of young childbearing. By the age of 17, for instance, 16 per cent of Bangladeshi wives have more than one child.[53] When unsafe abortion is used to end pregnancy arising too soon after childbirth, it introduces all of the risks of the procedure to a woman of reduced physical capacity to endure and recover from them.

4 *Parity (number of previous births)* Since pregnancy and childbirth in themselves present high health risks to women in many parts of the world, it follows that frequent pregnancy increases risks. Health may deteriorate progressively under the impact of repeated pregnancy, childbearing and childrearing, however, so that parity is a cumulative factor in reproductive health. It has been observed, for instance, that:

> At the Princess Christian Maternity Hospital in Sierra Leone, it is not unusual to see women who have brought 11 to 22 pregnancies to term. These women are usually very anaemic, and are exposed to such serious complications of pregnancy as postpartum haemorrhage, cord prolapse, and other hazards. Many reach the hospital with obstructed labour, infection and maternal exhaustion.[54]

Parity naturally tends to rise with age. In Botswana, for instance, women in the 45–49 year age group, in an urban area, have had on average six children, with five surviving, and seven, with six surviving in a rural area.[55] In Nigeria, grandmultiparity (four or more births) accounts for 17–21 per cent of all deliveries; women in West Africa have an average of 6.8 children.[56] In Jamaica, compared to women having their second child, those having their fifth to ninth births are 43 per cent more likely to die.[57] Similarly, evidence from rural Bangladesh shows that among women having their fourth or fifth birth, the risk of maternal death is almost double that of women having their second or third birth.[58]

5 *Limited access to reproductive health care* Women's access to reproductive health care is often limited for many reasons including poverty, illiteracy, spousal veto, and lack of availability of services in certain areas, including rural areas. Statistics cannot tell the real

stories of why women have limited access to services but they can indicate which women have limited access and are therefore at higher risk of maternal mortality. Statistics of maternal mortality, both in themselves and in relation to adolescence, advanced age and parity, sometimes distinguish urban from rural populations, and show the latter to be at a disadvantage.

For example, it has been shown that in the Ananthapur District in India 874 maternal deaths occur for every 100,000 live births in the rural area while 545 maternal deaths occur in the urban area.[59] This study indicates that some of the health service factors that lead to higher prevalence of maternal deaths in rural areas are lack of appropriately trained medical personnel, lack of transportation, and poor roads leading to the health service station.[60]

The rural setting renders delivery of health services more difficult and more expensive to achieve because widely distributed communities require time and travel to reach them. Medical equipment is often difficult to transport, and health centres equipped with adequate resources may be difficult for outlying peoples to reach, especially in an emergency. Health services, not only to save life endangered by advanced pregnancy and delivery but also to provide routine contraceptive care, may be simply inaccessible to rural residents of many countries.

Rural residence may deprive women both of reproductive care and of alternative lifestyles to early marriage and repeated pregnancy. It may also predispose them to early marriage and childbearing, and to multiparity. Urban life may offer inducements to postpone marriage and/or childbearing, through education and employment opportunities, and make a single woman's social and economic independence both possible and culturally acceptable. The fact of rural residence alone seems to impose a heavier toll on the health and the very lives of the women themselves and on the lives of their children.

6   *Abortion mortality* In England in 1937 the Birkett Committee was convened to study the abortion situation because it had been found that unskilled abortion, both self-induced and procured by unqualified practitioners, was an alarmingly frequent cause of women's deaths. In its Report, the Committee observed that the typical case of abortion involved a respectably married woman of modest income with two or more children who was seeking to terminate pregnancy to serve the best interests of her existing children and family.[61]

In many ways the health care circumstances of the English working classes in 1938 were comparable to the circumstances now prevailing in major population groups in the developing world. A retrospective analysis of 95 deaths due to abortion at Kenyatta National Hospital between 1974 and 1983 showed the average death rate to be nearly three deaths per 1,000 abortion admissions. The mean hospital stay was 12 days. Septic abortion with its complications accounted for 97.4 per cent of the deaths from induced abortion.[62]

Unskilled abortion is the leading cause of obstetric death in many parts of the world including Bangladesh, Columbia and Ethiopia.[63] Whilst the legalisation of abortion is a necessary first step in the reduction of abortion mortality it is not sufficient.[64] For abortion mortality to be significantly reduced, abortion services with appropriately trained health personnel and with contraceptive aftercare need to be made widely available, particularly to women, such as rural women, whose access to services is problematic. India changed its abortion law in 1971 to allow abortion for extended reasons. About 80 per cent of the Indian population live in rural areas where appropriately trained health personnel who can deliver such services are scarce. As a result 13 per cent of maternal deaths in rural India in 1980 were due to unskilled abortion.[65]

Human rights applicable to women's reproductive health

When the modern world tackled the task of reconstructing itself after 1945, it emphasized the need for respect for both human rights and individual health. The Preamble to the Charter[66] mandates the United Nations (UN) to promote solutions of health problems, which have international repercussions where both endemic and epidemic diseases are concerned. By Article 56 all members of the UN pledge themselves to joint and separate action in cooperation with the UN for the achievement of this purpose. Under Article 57, specialized agencies shall be established to work with the UN. Accordingly, WHO and, for instance, the United Nations Fund for Population Activities (UNFPA) have human rights responsibilities regarding women's survival and health. In order to recognize that international human rights protect not only communities but also each individual, the UN adopted the Universal Declaration of Human Rights.[67]

The Universal Declaration of Human Rights, approved without dissent by the United Nations General Assembly in 1948, was intended to be given effect in a Universal Covenant on Human Rights. In the course of drafting the Covenant it was decided to present its implementing provisions in separate instruments, one covering civil and political rights and the other dealing with economic, social and cultural rights.[68] The international instruments of primary interest in the analysis of the right of women to survive pregnancy and childbirth and the duty not to neglect women are the Covenant on Civil and Political Rights[69] and the Covenant on Economic, Social and Cultural Rights,[70] subsequently reinforced by the Convention on the Elimination of All Forms of Discrimination Against Women.[71]

At the regional level a number of human rights conventions exist which are relevant to women's reproductive survival. The European Convention on Human Rights and Fundamental Freedoms,[72] the American Convention on Human Rights[73] and the African Charter on Human and People's Rights all prohibit discrimination on the basis of sex.[74]

At a higher level of abstraction these international and regional human rights instruments contain expressions of the normative concept of human dignity.[75] The first Article of the Universal Declaration itself observes that '[a]ll human beings are born free and equal in dignity and rights'. These Human Rights Conventions pursue dignity through rights. Women's claims to human dignity are of special concern where they face the prospect of death from pregnancy and childbirth which can be prevented through provision of reproductive health care. Observance of the duty to provide such care is a minimum condition of civilized conduct, and the minimum tribute to human dignity.

The right to life

The most obvious human right violated by avoidable maternal death is the right to life itself. Whilst self-evident, the principle deserves to be expressed, and opens the way to consideration not only of the fact of life but also of the proper quality of life described as health. According to Article 6.1 of the Political Covenant, '[e]very human being has the inherent right to life. This right shall be protected by law. No one shall be arbitrarily deprived of his life.' In the traditions of the common law and other legal systems, a 'human being' is one who is in being by virtue of live birth.[76] This Article reflects Article 3 of the Universal Declaration: '[e]veryone has the right to life, liberty and security of the person.'

It is clear from the language of the latter, however, and from the context in which it appears, that the Article is directed towards judicial imposition of capital punishment.[77] The concern of both Articles is more with ensuring due process of law as a condition of a state's terminating an offender's life than with the absolute preservation of life itself. Assertions of the right to life are circumscribed by this historical context, and it may appear innovative to claim that the right entitles women to access to reproductive health care directed to their survival.

An important controversy with more than theoretical implications centres upon the scope of Article 6 of the Political Covenant quoted in part above: authorities disagree on whether it is to be given a narrow or a broad application. The right itself is not all-embracing. It is recognized that the right in itself 'does not guarantee any person against death from famine or cold or lack of medical attention'.[78] Accordingly, lack of costly obstetric services does not violate the right to life of a woman who requires such services to survive; there is no duty to apply unavailable or grossly disproportionate resources.[79]

Dinstein proposes a narrow reading of article 6: '[f]ailure to reduce infant mortality is not within Article 6, while practising or tolerating infanticide would violate the article'.[80] Opposing this view and advocating a much broader application is Ramcharan who finds that 'such a restrictive approach is no longer adequate and is contradicted by the available evidence of practice.'[81] The Human Rights Committee, established under the Political Covenant takes a broad approach to the right to life, which it considers to have been too narrowly interpreted. The Committee considers it desirable that States Parties to the Covenant take positive measures to reduce mortality by implementing measures to eliminate malnutrition and epidemics.[82]

It may be a requirement of Article 6 of the Political Covenant that a governmental decision to withhold resources from such programmes as family planning be conscientiously determined. Such programmes are of established effectiveness in avoiding calculable numbers of maternal deaths. By providing that '[n]o one shall be *arbitrarily* deprived of his life' (emphasis added) Article 6 suggests that cost-effective family planning programme should not be withheld, terminated or underfunded by governmental neglect or capriciousness.[83] Maine and her colleagues explained that the least expensive programme options of:

1   providing first aid at a health centre with transportation of the most serious cases to a small, nearby hospital
2   obstetric first aid at health centres; and/or
3   averting high-risk and unwanted pregnancies through family planning programmes

would cost roughly US $2,600 per maternal death averted.[84] They estimate that other programme options depending on the services involved could range in cost between US $8,000 to US $42,000 per death averted.[85] Choosing among the programme options to determine the most cost-effective way to reduce maternal mortality would require analysis of the obstetrics, health service and reproductive factors in each individual community. The authors suggest that a decentralized approach might be the most cost-effective.[86]

It may be seriously contended that every country at risk of having high levels of maternal mortality is obliged to have and maintain appropriate preventive and remedial programmes. The burden is upon any country lacking an apparently competent programme to explain and justify its absence and show that it is neither arbitrary nor negligent.

The right to health care

There is no more a right to be healthy than there is a right to be tall. However, a woman may reasonably claim an entitlement at least to appropriate reproductive health care so as to enable her to survive pregnancy and childbirth. Women may claim a right to such health services as are achievable within the economic and social circumstances of their nations.

Although implicit in the right to life, the right to health care has independent content in international law. The Economic Covenant recognizes in Article 12.1 'the right of everyone to the enjoyment of the highest attainable standard of physical and mental health'. It obliges states to use their health resources according to utilitarian ideals.[87] This right to the 'highest attainable standard' health in line with the WHO Constitution, equates to 'a state of complete physical, mental and social well-being and not merely the absence of disease or infirmity'.[88] A definition of health itself, however, cannot easily serve as a programme to redress social inequity, or to relieve idiosyncratic disadvantage. From the perspective of international human rights law, therefore, it may be necessary to conceptualize an individual's health rather as the absence of preventable disease or infirmity.

Primary responsibility for achieving 'the highest attainable standard' rests with WHO. In formulating its policies WHO has developed the approach of primary health care.[89] The fundamental concept of this approach is that:

> Primary health care is essential health care based on practical, scientifically sound and socially acceptable methods and technology made universally accessible to individuals and families in the community through their full participation and at a cost that the community and country can afford to maintain at every stage of their development in the spirit of self reliance and self determination. It forms an integral part both of the country's health system, of which it is the central

function and main focus, and of the overall social economic development of the community. It is the first level of contact of individuals, the family and community with a national health system bringing health care as close as possible to where people live and work, and constitutes the first element of a continuing health care process.[90]

This approach, further developed in WHO's Global Strategy for Health for All by the Year 2000, suggests that 5 per cent of the gross national product of a country should be allocated to health[91] and a reasonable percentage of the health care expenditure be devoted to primary health care.[92] It further suggests that primary health care be made available to the whole population and suggests that it contains at least the following:

- safe water in the home or within 15 minutes walking distance, and adequate sanitary facilities in the home or immediate vicinity;
- immunization against diphtheria, tetanus, whooping cough, measles, poliomyelitis and tuberculosis;
- trained personnel for attending pregnancy and childbirth and caring for children up to at least 1 year of age.[93]

WHO's Seventh General Programme of Work (1984–89) specifies that at least two-thirds of births have to be attended by trained health workers.[94] However, in several African countries only 20–40 per cent of deliveries were attended by trained health workers.[95] A WHO Tabulation of Coverage of Maternity Care shows wide variations in percentages of births covered by trained attendants.[96] In Mali 14 per cent of births were assisted by trained attendants in 1981;[97] in Somalia it was 2 per cent in 1983;[98] in Syria it was 12 per cent in the rural area in 1979;[99] in India a year before it was 24 per cent in the rural areas;[100] and in Honduras as a whole it was 34 per cent in 1977.[101]

In addition to the Strategy for Health for All by the Year 2000, there is also the Nairobi Forward-Looking Strategies for the Advancement of Women which states:

Considering the unacceptably high levels of maternal mortality in many developing countries, the reduction of maternal mortality from now to the year 2000 to a minimum . . . level should be a key target for governments and nongovernmental organizations, including professional organizations.[102]

Unfortunately neither the Strategy for Health for All nor the Nairobi Forward-Looking Strategies sets a standard for the reduction of maternal mortality to a specific level. The Global Health Strategies does this for infant mortality by requiring all WHO members to reduce infant death rates to 50 per 1000 live births by the year 2000.[103] The fact that such an absolute goal has not been set for the reduction of maternal mortality indicates that health officials know little of the extent of the problem due in part to lack of death registration in many countries.[104]

WHO's Eighth Central Programme of Work will no doubt reflect in a more specific way Dr Mahler's call for action to reduce maternal mortality by half in the next decade. It would be a minimum tribute to women and their families for countries to reallocate their budgets to focus their health resources on reduction of maternal mortality and morbidity. Given 'the right of everyone to the enjoyment of the highest attainable standard of physical and mental health',[105] the demonstrably inappropriate use of scarce resources is arguably illegal, not merely unwise.

The right to found a family

An international human right which is especially dependent on women's survival is the right to found a family. In addition to serving human dignity, this right is compatible with prohibitions of genocide and of sex discrimination. Article 23 of the Political Covenant is representative of several other Conventions[106] in providing that:

1   The family is the natural and fundamental group unit of society and is entitled to protections by society and the State.
2   The right of men and women of marriageable age to marry and to found a family shall be recognized.

Such language shows that the protected right is not just to give birth, but to establish and raise a family. The right is necessarily dependent on women's right to life, but also their right to their families: absence of appropriate services may violate both rights.

Article 16(10 (e)) of the Women's Convention[107] amplifies the content of this right by obligating States Parties to ensure men and women:

> The same rights to decide freely and responsibly on the number and spacing of their children and to have access to the information, education and means to enable them to exercise these rights.

The right to found a family embraces not simply a right to conceive, bear and rear children, but the right of a woman to maximize her chances of surviving childbirth – for instance, by delaying her first birth – and her right to space births so as to maximize her children's chances of survival. That is, she must have the 'means' to found a family of her preferred size without undue repetition of pregnancy to compensate for lost children. As a practical matter, the duty to implement this right is discharged in part through the provision of family planning and basic obstetric services and the 'information' and 'education' necessary to use these services.

The right to sexual nondiscrimination

Transcending specific rights under leading human rights conventions is the generic right to equality of both sexes to enjoyment of all rights. Article 3 of the Political Covenant provides that:

> The States Parties to the present Covenant 'undertake' to ensure the equal rights of men and women to the enjoyment of all civil and political rights set forth in the present Covenant.

Article 3 of the Economic Covenant provides that States Parties undertake the same regarding the enjoyment of all economic, social and cultural rights which this Covenant sets forth.

The entire Women's Convention is self-evidently dedicated to equality of the sexes and its Article 1 defines 'discrimination against women' to mean:

> . . . any distinction, exclusion or restriction made on the basis of sex which has the effect or purpose of impairing or nullifying the recognition, enjoyment or exercise by women, irrespective of their marital status, on a basis of equality of men and women, of human rights and fundamental freedoms in the political, economic, social, cultural, civil or any other field.

Differential treatment of women which results in unwanted pregnancy, or disadvantages to their health constitutes 'discrimination against women'. Article 12 (1) of the Women's Convention provides that:

> States Parties shall take all appropriate measures to eliminate discriminations against women in the field of health care in order to ensure, on a basis of equality of men and women, access to health care services, including those related to family planning.

As a result, States Parties have to repeal laws and policies, such as rules which condition women's – but not men's – access to health care and family planning services, and which have the effect of denying women their rights.

There are many examples of requirements which inhibit equal access to health care and family planning services.[108] In some countries, husbands, but not wives, are allowed to obtain contraceptives without spousal authorization; in others, unmarried men, but not unmarried women, may obtain contraceptive services.[109] In some countries voluntary sterilization services are available only to women for therapeutic reasons but not to men, thus discriminating against men in denying men equal access to such services.[110]

In determining whether such requirements, for example spousal veto of family planning services, constitute discrimination against women, two questions must be asked:

1 Do spousal veto practices make 'any distinction, exclusion, or restriction' on the basis of sex?
2 If they do make a distinction, does it have 'the effect or purpose of impairing or nullifying the recognition, enjoyment or exercise by women, irrespective of their marital status, on a basis of equality of men and women, of human rights and fundamental freedoms. . . .'?[111]

The answer to the first question is 'yes'. Where a spousal veto can be exercised by the husband but not the wife, there is a 'distinction' on the basis of sex on the face of the law, policy, or guideline in question. Where the law provides for a veto power for both husband and wife but a clinic applies it in such a way as to recognize only the husband's power of veto, a restriction on women is made in the way the law is applied.

The answer to the second question is also affirmative. Spousal veto practices have 'the effect or purpose of impairing or nullifying' women's recognition or exercise of their human rights or freedoms.[112]

This same analysis can be used to show discrimination against men – for example in denying men, but not women, access to voluntary sterilization. Where laws or clinic practices limit men's access to family planning services,[113] it is important to argue for their repeal because any form of sex discrimination, whether against men or women, can be used as a rationale for additional forms of sex discrimination. Once it is established that sex discrimination, whether against men or women, violates a person's human rights, that decision can be used to argue against other discriminatory practices rooted in the same basis.

Enforcement

International human rights conventions impose legal duties not to neglect women's lives and health. Duties arising under these conventions are owed according to the general principles of international treaty law[114] to other States Parties, to other signatories and to agencies created by individual conventions for their enforcement.[115] Further, covenants may themselves oblige States Parties to implement them in their domestic law.[116] Whilst the enforcement of international treaty obligations in municipal courts is governed by the jurisprudence of individual countries,[117] many domestic tribunals will find that duties do exist to observe basic human rights. They may come directly from international conventions, or indirectly through national constitutions or, for instance, human rights codes, interpretation of which may be influenced by presumptions that countries intend in good faith to give effect to their international commitments, and that they do not intend that their municipal laws should violate them.[118]

Domestic enforcement

Article 2 of the Political Covenant and the Economic Covenant and the Women's Convention requires States Parties to implement the recognized rights by means, *inter alia*, of domestic legislation. Further, whilst the Economic Covenant and the Women's Convention rely upon 'progressive implementation' achieved over a period of time,[119] the Political Covenant appears to impose in principle an immediate obligation to ensure observance of its requirements, taking into account only 'the need in some cases for time to adapt national legislation to the Covenant's requirements'.[120] The obligation to enact legislative protection of treaties' rights is residual in the sense that, in some cases, other domestic legal provisions such as in constitutions,[121] court judgements and earlier legislation may give adequate protection; so may administrative measures and constitutional conventions (although these latter means may be less legally secure).

The Political Covenant employs more explicit language than the Economic Covenant or the Women's Convention in obliging each State Party 'to ensure to all individuals within its territory and subject to its jurisdiction the rights recognized' in the Covenant.[122] The obligation is an 'obligation of result'[123] in that States Parties are obliged to take measures necessary 'to give effect to the rights recognized' in the Covenant[124] through means of their own selection. The obligation to ensure rights includes an obligation to ensure enforcement of effective remedies[125] ' . . . determined by competent judicial, administrative or legislative authorities, or by any other competent authority provided for by the legal system of the state' and to develop the possibilities of judicial remedy.[126] The remedy shall be granted 'notwithstanding that the violation has been committed by persons acting in an official capacity.'[127]

Reliance upon domestic procedures for the prevention and remedy of legal violations may place some at a disadvantage even though the disadvantage may reflect historic purposes of protection. In particular, women in some legal systems may lack individual procedural capacity, and others claiming to act on their behalf – such as husbands – may have to meet special legal qualifications. There is frequent evidence, however, that the incidence of mortality is highest among those who are least advantaged economically, educationally, socially and otherwise, and it seems improbable that such disadvantaged women will pursue substantive claims against their governments in order to assert their rights.

Domestic enforcement may often depend, therefore, upon public officers, such as ombudsmen and women's advocates, and upon national organizations and branches of international organizations. Indeed, countries may discharge their duty to ensure enforcement of remedies in part by appointing public officers to act on behalf of women through judicial and administrative channels and by, for instance, representing particular injured or deceased women in pursuit of compensatory remedies, or seeking preventive remedies on behalf of women, both in particular and in general. Their social and political advocacy may include urging implementation of reproductive health care programmes.

The Political Covenant does not specify the nature of the remedy required in response to a violated right. This raises both substantive and procedural difficulties. Class actions may make more impact than private claims, but they are rarely accommodated under procedural rules as liberal as those in force in the USA.[128] Public relief such as a judicial declaration may be of political significance but, in that it carries no enforcement, it may not constitute a 'remedy'.

The legal rights enforceable in municipal courts may not be individual rights to a substantive outcome, but procedural rights to have human rights claims properly determined. Women, for instance, may not have a legal right to the provision of reproductive health services, but they may have a right to have their claim upon health resources determined fairly and without discrimination on such grounds as sex. Further, one may recognize a duty among States Parties to give effect to human rights conventions conscientiously, to allocate resources to basic health needs and not to invoke special grounds, such as national emergency, in prioritizing competing interests.[129] It must be doubted, however, whether municipal courts would direct governments on priorities; equivalents of the Act of State Doctrine may render resource allocation issues non-justiciable, leaving them to the political arena.

The means of pursuing domestic remedies are important not only in themselves, but because their exhaustion is usually a precondition to presentation of a claim at an international level. International legal doctrine has the experience and sense of reality not to require exhaustion of local remedies where in fact no substantive remedies exist, despite their theoretical availability.[130] Accordingly, a government which frustrates plaintiffs' attempts to pursue local remedies by operation of substantive, procedural or administrative barriers, may be found to have created a jurisdiction in which no local remedies in fact exist. The matter will then qualify for presentation, pursuit and remedy at the international level.

International enforcement

Contemporary commentaries on the Covenants and the Women's Convention make clear their different means of potential enforcement.[131] The Human Rights Committee, established by the Political Covenant[132] is to receive reports by States Parties on the measures they have adopted which give effect to rights recognized in the Covenant and on the progress made in exercise of those rights. The reports are transmitted to the Committee by the UN Secretary-General.[133] The Committee can also receive communications from States Parties claiming that another State Party is not fulfilling its obligations under the Covenant.[134] The Committee will consider such communications only if local remedies have been exhausted.[135] The Committee must make every attempt at conciliation of the States Parties concerned and may appoint an *ad hoc* Conciliation Commission.[136]

The Committee also has the power under the Optional Protocol to the Covenant[137] to receive communications from individuals regarding a State Party to the Protocol.[138] The Committee will consider a communication from an individual only if that individual has exhausted local remedies and if the matter is not being examined by another international body.[139] It will examine the communication, forward its views to the State Party and the individual[140] and include its activities in its annual report.[141]

Implementation of the Economic Covenant and the Women's Convention requires States Parties to report respectively to the Economic, Social and Cultural Committee, established by the Economic and Social Council (ECOSOC),[142] and the Committee on the Elimination of Discrimination Against Women established under the Women's Convention,[143] the measures they have adopted and the progress they have made in achieving the observance of the respective Covenant rights.[144] These reports to the Economic Committee may also be sent by ECOSOC to the UN Commission on Human Rights.[145] The reports shall be sent to the UN Secretary General, whose duty it is to transmit copies to ECOSOC,[146] and to the relevant UN specialized agencies.[147] ECOSOC and the Commission may report their recommendations on economic, social and cultural rights to the UN General Assembly but they may not make specific observations, comments or recommendations on the record of any specific country.[148]

It has been noted that specialized agencies 'have a fundamental responsibility to promote realization of human rights', and that 'the primary thrust of the [Political Covenant's] implementation procedure is directed at the agencies'.[149] The role of agencies, such as WHO and UNFPA, is particularly credible because of their access to national data and their capacity to make assessments of the most cost-effective health interventions. From such sources they may attempt to create standards required to be observed which are inspired by a vision of the ideal but predicated upon knowledge of the achievable. In this sense, such agencies can monitor performance under the Covenant and protect its values. Specialized agencies can also acquire national data and produce estimates of maternal mortality due to absence of health services.

The existing work of WHO, particularly its Global Strategy for Health for All by the Year 2000, is notable, and furnishes materials through which the substance of standards may be fashioned. WHO might usefully work with the Human Rights Committee, the Economic Social and Cultural Committee and Committee on the Elimination of Discrimination Against Women to apply the indicators developed for the Global Strategy to those aspects of reports of States Parties under the respective human rights treaties concerned with maternal survival and health.[150] Where proven strategies have been publicized to meet internationally agreed goals for achievement, countries declining or failing to apply them may be called to legal account, under the respective Covenants and, for example, the Women's Convention.

Beneath the formal and informal functions of international agencies operate a number of prominent non-governmental organizations such as International Planned Parenthood Federation and regional and national voluntary organizations. Their legal powers before international and national tribunals may be modest,[151] but they may enjoy influence beyond their formal power. They may monitor national performances, publicize deficiencies in national achievements, and press for improvements with respect to national health and survival.

Conclusion

International law has evolved in recent decades to restrain governments from actively abusing their citizens. The challenge ahead is to extend human rights to prevent governments from passively abusing the life and health of their citizens – particularly their female citizens – by neglect. The task of establishing a legally constituted human right to women's reproductive health requires establishment of legal duties to service that right.

Notes

1   World Health Organization, *Prevention of Maternal Mortality: A Report of a WHO Interregional Meeting*, 1985, p. 5.
2   Mahler, H., 'The safe motherhood initiative: a call to action, **668** *The Lancet* 21 March 1987, speech given at the International 'Safe Motherhood' Conference, Nairobi, 10–13 February 1987.
3   Hartfield, V. J., 'Maternal mortality in Nigeria compared with earlier international experience', **18**(1) *International Journal of Gynecology and Obstetrics* 1980, p. 70. Schofield, R., 'Did mothers really die? Three centuries of maternal mortality in the world we have lost' in Bonfield, L., Smith, R. M. and Wrightson, K. (eds), *The World We Have Gained: Histories of Population and Social Structure*, Oxford, Basil Blackwell, 1986.
4   See generally Davies, M. L. (ed.), *Maternity: Letters from Working Women*, New York and London, Norton and Co., 1915 (reprinted 1978).
5   Strachey, R., 'The prison house of home' in *The Cause: Short History of the Women's Movement in Great Britain*, 11, London, Virago, 1929 (reprinted 1979).
6   See generally, Fortney, J. A., 'The importance of family planning in reducing maternal mortality', **18**(2) *Studies in Family Planning*, 1987, 109.
7   See, generally, Maine, D. and McNamara, R., *Birth Spacing and Child Survival*, New York, Centre for Population and Family Health, Columbia University, 1985.
8   See generally, Maine, D., *Family Planning: Its Impact on the Health of Women and Children*, New York, Centre for Population and Family Health, Columbia University, 1982.
9   Ibid., pp. 9, 25.
10   *Bravery* v. *Bravery* [1954] 3 All ER 59 at pp. 67–8.
11   *Royal College of Nursing of the United Kingdom* v. *Department of Health and Social Security* [1981] 1 All ER 545.
12   Ibid., p. 556.
13   Ibid., p. 563.
14   See, generally, Cook, R. J. and Dickens, B. M., *Issues in Reproductive Health Law in the Commonwealth*, London, Commonwealth Secretariat, 1986.
15   World Health Organization, *Maternal Mortality Rates: A Tabulation of Available Information*, 2, 1986.

16 Fortney, *loc cit.*, note 6, *supra*.
17 Id.
18 Ibid., p. 110.
19 Ibid.
20 Ibid., p. 111.
21 Ibid., p. 112.
22 Rosenfield, A. and Maine, D., 'Maternal mortality. A neglected tragedy', **446**(2) *The Lancet*, 1985, p. 83.
23 WHO, note 15, *supra*.
24 Ibid., p. 3.
25 Id.
26 Id.
27 WHO note 1, *supra.*, at p. 4.
28 Id.
29 See explanation of causes in Dr M. Fathalla's description of a 'woman's road to death' in WHO note 1, *supra*, at p. 5.
30 Note 2, *supra*.
31 See generally for fuller explanation of such factors, Maine, D., Rosenfield, A., Wallace, M., Kimball, A., Kwast, B., Papiernik, E. and White, S., *Prevention of Maternal Deaths in Developing Countries: Program Options and Practical Considerations*, Background Paper prepared for the International 'Safe Motherhood' Conference, Nairobi, 10–13, February 1987 pp. 4–12, available fromD. Maine, Centre for Population and Family Health, School of Public Health, Columbia University, 60 Haven Avenue, New York, NY 10032.
32 Ibid., p. 4.
33 Ibid., p. 5.
34 Note 2, *supra*, p. 670.
35 Note 1, *supra* at p. 6.
36 Ibid., p. 7
37 Note 31 *supra.*, p. 10.
38 Id.
39 Id.
40 See generally, 'Healthier mothers and children through family planning', *Population Reports*, The Johns Hopkins University Population Information Program, Series J. no. 27, 1984.
41 Manyenang, W. G., Khulamani, P., Larson, M. K. and Wayu, A. A., *Botswana Family Health Survey 1985*, 1985 p. 111, available from Contraceptive Prevalence Survey Program, Westinghouse Public Applied Systems, P.O. Box 866. Columbia Md. 21044, USA.
42 See 'Digest', **11**(3) *Int'l. Family Planning Perspectives*, 1985, 98, summarizing National Population Bureau, *The Nigeria Fertility Survey 1981/1982, Principal Report*, 1984.
43 Paxman, J. M. and Zuckerman, R. J., *Laws and Policies Affecting Adolescent Health 98* Geneva, WHO 1987.
44 1d.
45 In the Carribean, for example, it is common practice that pregnant schoolgirls leave school with no chance for re-admission (McKay, J. (ed.), *Adolescent Fertility: Report of International Consultation 1983*); International Planned Parenthood Federation cited in Cook and Dickens op. cit., note 14, *supra* at p. 25.
46 Wanjala, S., Murugu, N., and Mati, J., 'Mortality due to abortion at Kenyatta National Hospital, 1974–1983' in Ciba Foundation Symposium *Abortion: Medical Progress and Social Implications*, London, Pitman, 1985, p. 44.

47 'Youth in the 1980's: social and health concerns', *Population Reports*, Series M, no. 9, 1985, p. 365.
48 Id.
49 Chen, L. C., Gsche, M. C. *et al.*, 'Maternal mortality in rural Bangladesh', 5(11) *Studies in Family Planning* 1974, 334.
50 Note 1 *supra*, at p. 7.
51 Note 8 *supra* at p. 30.
52 On average, in the developing world, 1 in 5 infant deaths could be averted if births were spaced more than two years apart: note 7 supra, at p. 17.
53 Petros-Barvazian, A., 'Family planning: A preventive health measure', **57** *Journal of the Christian Medical Association of India*, 1984.
54 See *Meeting the Needs of the 80's*, Report of the 5th Int'l Conference on Voluntary Surgical Contraception, World Federation of Health Agencies for the Advancement of Voluntary Surgical Contraception, 1985, p. 5.
55 Manyeneng *et al.*, op. cit., note 41 *supra*, at p. 95.
56 See Report of Conference on Reproductive Health Management in Sub-Saharan Africa, November 1984. Abstract of paper by A. E. Omu. No. 28, available from the World Federation of Health Agencies for the Advancement of Voluntary Surgical Contraception, 122 East 42nd Street, New York, NY 10168.
57 Note 1 *supra*, at p. 7.
58 Note 49 *supra*.
59 Bhatia, J., 'Maternal mortality in Ananthapur District, India: preliminary findings of a study', WHO Doc. no. FHE/PMM. B5.9.16 cited in Maine, *et al. loc. cit.*, note 31, *supra*.
60 Bhatia, J., 'Maternal mortality in Ananthapur District, Andrha Pradesh, India', Indian Institute of Management, Bangalore, September 1986, cited in Maine, *et al.*, *loc. cit.*, note 31, *supra*, at p. 12.
61 UK Government, *Report of the Inter-Departmental Committee on Abortion* (chaired by Norman Birkett) 1939, cited in Dickens, B. M., *Abortion and the Law*, London, McGibbon and Kee, 1966, p. 13.
62 Note 46 *supra*, p. 41.
63 Note 1 *supra*, p. 6; see generally 'Complications of abortion in the developing world' *Population Reports*, Series F, no. 7, 1980, p. 109.
64 See, generally, Cook, R. J. And Dickens, B. M., 'A decade of international change in abortion law: 1967–1977', **68**(7) *American Journal of Public Health* 1978; Tietze, C. and Henshaw, S., *Induced Abortion: A World View 1986*, New York, The Alan Guttmacher Institute, 1986.
65 Bahl Dhall, S., 'Training and delivery of abortion in India', in Landy, U. and Ratnam, S. S. (eds), *Prevention and Treatment of Contraceptive Failure*, New York, Plenum Press, p. 73.
66 Charter of the United Nations *signed* 26 June 1945, *entered into force* 24 October 1945, 59 Stat. 1031, TS no. 993, 3 Bevans 1153 (1969).
67 Universal Declaration of Human Rights, BA res. 217A(111), UN Doc. A/N10, at 71(1948) [hereinafter referred to as the Universal Declaration].
68 Sohn, *The Short History of United Nations Documents on Human Rights*, in *The United Nations and Human Rights*, 37, 169 (Commission to Study the Organization of Peace 1968).
69 International Covenant on Civil and Political Rights *adopted* 19 December 1966, *entered into force* 23 March 1976, G(A) Res. 2200 (XXI) 21 UN GADR Supp. (No. 16) 52 UN Doc. A/6316 (1966) [hereinafter referred to as Politicial Covenant].
70 International Covenant on Economic, Social and Cultural Rights, *adopted* 19 December, 1966, *entered into force* 3 January 1976, GA Res. 2200 (XXI), 21 UN

GADR, Supp. (no. 16) 49, Doc. A/6316 (1966). [hereinafter referred to as the Economic Covenant].

71 The Convention on the Elimination of All Forms of Discrimination Against Women, *adopted* 18 December 1979, *entered into force* 3 September 1981, GA Res 34/180 (xxxiv), 34 UN GADR Supp. (no. 46) at 193, Doc. A/39/45. [hereinafter referred to as the Women's Convention)

72 European Convention on Human Rights, *adopted* 4 November 1950, *entered into force* 3 September 1953, 213 UNTS 222, Article 14.

73 American Convention on Human Rights, *adopted* 22 November 1969, *entered into force* 28 July 1978, OAS Treaty Series no. 36 at 1, Article 1.

74 African Charter on Human and People's Rights, *adopted* 27 June 1981, *entered into force* 21 October, 1986, OAU Doc DAB/:EG/67/3 Rev. 5 reprinted in 21 ILM 58 (1982), Article 2.

75 Schacter, 'Editorial comment . . . Human dignity as a normative concept', **77** *AJTL* 1983, 48.

76 The words 'everyone' and 'human being', have been authoritatively interpreted by domestic and international human rights judicial tribunals to be limited to children from birth. In the case upholding the legality of the abortion provision of the Reform Act of the Austrian Penal Code (Federal Law 23 January 1974), the Austrian Constitutional Court interpreted Article 2 on the right to life of the [European] Convention for the Protection of Human Rights and Fundamental Freedoms not to protect unborn life. In *Paton v. United Kingdom* 3 EHRR 408 (1980), the European Commission interpreted the same Article 2 consistently with the Austrian Constitutional Court. The Inter-American Commission considered for the first time the scope of Article 1 on the right to life of the American Declaration of the Rights and Duties of Man. This Commission found that the US abortion law as articulated in *Roe v. Wade* 410 US 113(1973) does not violate Article 1 of the Declaration.

77 See generally, Sieghart, P., *The International Law of Human Rights*, Oxford, Clarendon Press, 1983, pp. 126–34.

78 Robinson, N., *The Universal Declaration of Human Rights: its Origins, Significance and Interpretation*, (2nd edn.), New York, Institute of Jewish Affairs, 1958, p. 106.

79 Pope Pius XII emphasized obligations relevant to ordinary means of medical treatment at 1957 international congress of anaesthesiologists: 'Morally one is held to use ordinary means – according to circumstances of persons, places, times and cultures – that is to say, means that do not involve any grave burden for oneself or another. A more strict obligation would be too burdensome for most men and would render the attachment of the higher, more important good too difficult. Life, health, all temporal activities are in fact subordinated to spiritual ends. On the other hand, one is not forbidden to take more than the strictly necessary steps to preserve life and health, as long as he does not fail in some more serious duty.': 'The Pope speaks: prolongation of life', 4 *Obseratore Romano* 1957, 393–98.

80 Dinstein, 'The right to life, physical integrity and liberty' in Henkin, L. (ed.), *The International Bill of Rights: The Covenant on Civil and Political Rights*, New York, Columbia University Press, pp. 114, 116; see also Ramcharan, B. G. (ed), *The Right to Life in International Law*, London, Kluwer, 1985.

81 Ramcharan, B. G., 'The concept and dimensions of the right to life' in Ramcharan, op. cit., note 80 *supra*, pp. 1,4.

82 Ibid., p. 5.

83 State liability for gross negligence for failure to pursue known offenders was found and damages were awarded in the Janes Case (1926) by the United

States–Mexico General Claims Commission, Annual Digest of Public International Law Cases, 1925–26, no. 158. 70.

84 Note 31 supra, at 28.

85 Id.

86 Ibid., p. 33.

87 On the drafting history of Article 12 and on related European Conventions, see ROSCAN-ABBING, *International Organizations in Europe and the Right to Health Care*, London, Kluwer, 1979, p. 64.

88 The Preamble to the Constitution of the World Health Organization, **3** *Official Records of the World Health Organization* June 1948, p. 100.

89 *World Health Organization, Primary Health Care*, Report of the International Conference on Primary Health Care (Alma Ata USSR, 6–12 September, 1978) 'Health for All Series' no. 1.

90 Ibid., part VI, at p. 3.

91 Global indicator 4, *World Health Organization, Global Strategies for Health For All by the Year 2000*, Health for All Series, no. 3, 1981, p. 75.

92 Ibid.; Global Indicator 4, *Evaluation of the Strategy For Health For All by the Year 2000; Seventh Report on the World Health Situation*, 1986, p. 50, indicates that some regions are noticeably better in achieving this goal. For example, 18 of the 23 countries in WHO's Latin American Region in contrast to only 5 of the 19 countries in WHO's Eastern Mediterranean Region spent 5 per cent of their GNP on health.

93 Global Indicator, note 91, *supra*.

94 *World Health Organization, Seventh General Programme of Work 1984–1989*, Health for All Series no. 8, 83, 1982.

95 Note 92, supra, at 38.

96 See, generally, WHO *Coverage of Maternity Care: A Tabulation of Available Information*, 1985.

97 Ibid., p. 8.

98 Ibid., p. 10.

99 Ibid., p. 17

100 Ibid., p. 18.

101 Ibid., p. 13.

102 *Forward-Looking Strategies of Implementation for the Advancement of Women and Concrete Measures to Overcome Obstacles to the Achievement of the Goals and Objectives of the United Nations Decade for Women for the Period 1986 to the Year 2000: Equality, Development and Peace*. A/Con. 116/28/Rev. 1, 1985.

103 Indicator 9, note 91 *supra*, at 76.

104 Note 2 *supra*, p. 668.

105 Art. 12.1, Economic Covenant, note 70 *supra*

106 Note 102 *supra*; also note 72 *supra*, 7, 199–200.

107 See Cook, R. J. and Haws, J. M., 'The United Nations Convention on the Rights of Women: opportunities for family planning providers', **12**(2) *International Family Planning Perspective*, 1986, 49.

108 Ibid., p. 50–2.

109 Ibid.

110 Cock and Haws, 'The UN Convention on the Rights of Women', op. cit., p. 50, see generally Foss, J. A., Hong, S. and Huber, D., *Voluntary Sterilization: An International Fact Book*, New York, Association for Voluntary Surgical Contraception, 1985, pp. 17–21.

111 Cook, R. J. and Maine, D., 'Spousal veto over family planning services' **77**(3) *American Journal of Public Health* 1987, 339.

112 Note 111, supra, pp. 340–1.

113 Note 107, *supra*, p. 50 and note 111, *supra*, p. 341.

114 See the Vienna Convention on the Law of Treaties, *adopted* 23 May 1969, *entered into force* 27 January 1980, UN Doc. A/CONF. 39/27 (1969), reprinted in 63 AJIL 875(1969), B ILM 679(1969).

115 Regarding the international enforcement of the Political Covenant, see Robertson, 'The implementation system: international measures' in Henkin, op. cit., note 80 *supra*, p. 332.

116 Regarding the domestic enforcement of the Political Covenant, see Schacter, 'The obligation to implement the Covenant in Domestic Law', in Henkin, op. cit., note 80 *supra*, 311.

117 Brudner, 'The domestic enforcement of international covenants on human rights: a theoretical framework' 35 *Univeristy of Toronto Law Journal*, 1985, 219.

118 See note 92 supra, at p. 42 for examples of municipal legislation passed in support of the Global Health Strategy.

119 For discussion of the Principle of Progressive Realization, see Trubek, 'Economic, social and cultural rights in the Third World: human rights law and human needs programs' in Meron, T. (ed.), *Human Rights and International Law: Legal and Policy Issues*, Oxford, Clarendon, pp. 205, 213.

120 Schacter, 'The obligation to implement the Covenant in Domestic Law', in Henkin, *op. cit.*, note 80 *supra*, p. 324.

121 Many national constitutions have health care provisions; see for instance, the provision that:

It is an essential function of the State to look after the health of the people of the Republic. The individual, as part of the community, is entitled to the promotion, protection, conservation, restoration and recovery of his health, and has the obligation of preserving it. Health is understood as complete physical, mental and social well-being. (Constitution of Panama, Article 103.)

122 Art. 2(1) Political Covenant, note 69 *supra*.

123 *Schacter, loc. cit.*, note 120 *supra*.

124 Art. 2.2 Political Covenant, note 69 supra.

125 Ibid.; and Art. 2.3(b).

126 Id.

127 Art. 2.3(a). This provision 'was presumably intended to override a possible claim of official immunity'; see Schacter, *loc. cit.*, note 120 *supra*, p. 326.

128 See, generally, Ontario Law Reform Commission, *Report on Class Actions*, 1982.

129 *Greek Cases* [1968], Council of Europe, Eur. Comm., HR Decisions 25(1968) 116, *Gov. of Denmark* v. *Gov. of Greece*, App No. 3321/67, *Gov. of Norway* v. *Gov. of Greece*, App No. 3322/67, *Gov. of Sweden* v. *Gov. of Greece* App. No. 3323/67, *Gov. of the Netherlands* v. *Gov. of Greece* App No. 3344/67 (Decision 24 January 1968).

130 An individual is not required 'to exhaust justice where there is no justice to exhaust', Robert E. Brown case (*US* v. *UK*) (1923), RIAA, Vol. 6, 120, discussed in Brierly, J. L., *The Law of Nations; An Introduction to the International Law of Peace*, (6th edn. ed. by Waldock, H.,) 1963, p. 282.

131 See generally, Henkin, op. cit., note 80, *supra*; Trubek, note 119 *supra*, Burrows, N., 'The 1979 Convention on the Elimination of All Forms of Discrimination Against Women' 32 *Netherlands International Law Review* 1985, 419.

132 Art. 28, Political Covenant, note 69 *supra*.

133 Ibid., Art. 40.

134 Ibid., Art. 41.

135 Ibid., Art. 41 1(C)

136 Ibid., Art. 42
137 Optional Protocol to the International Covenant, on Civil and Political Rights, *adopted* 19 December 1966, *entered into force* 23 March, 1976, GA Res. 2200(XXI), 21 UN GADR, Supp. (No. 16) 59, UN Doc. A6316(1966).
138 Ibid., Art. 1. See communication No. R 9/35 submitted under this Optional Protocol by S. Aumeeruddy – Cziffra and 19 other Mauritian women successfully alleging sex discrimination.
139 Ibid., Art. 5.2(a) and (b).
140 Ibid., Art. 5.3, 5.4.
141 Ibid., Art. 6.
142 Art. 16(1) Economic Covenant, note 71 supra; ECOSOC recently established this Committee whose 18 members consist of individuals recognized for their expertise and competence in the field of human rights. UN ESCOR Supp. No. 1 at 15, UN Doc. E/RES/1985/17(1985).
143 Economic Covenant, note 71 supra, Art. 17.
144 Economic Covenant, Art. 16 note 71 *supra*.
145 Economic Covenant, note 71, supra, Art. 19.
146 Ibid., Art. 16.2(a).
147 Ibid., Art. 16.2(b).
148 Trubek, note 119 *supra*, at 218.
149 Alston, 'The United Nations' specialized agencies and implementation of the International Covenant on Economic, Social and Cultural Rights', **18** *Columbia Journal of Transnational Law*, 1979, 79, 117.
150 For example, the Indicators for Monitoring Progress Towards Health for All by the Year 2000 (1981) (note 102 *supra*) might be used by States Parties as guidelines for reporting under the Economic Covenant to make these reports more substantive rather than descriptive; see for an example of the descriptive approach, Report of Spain to ECOSOC on the Implementation of the Economic Covenant E/1986/4/Add. 6 27 January 1986.
151 But see the right of individual petition to the Human Rights Committee against States accepting the Optional Protocol to the Civil and Political Rights Covenants, note 141 *supra*.

9 Women, rights and reproduction

SHEILA MCLEAN

At first sight, it may seem striking that, in a book which is concerned with human reproduction, so much of the discussion concentrates on issues which might be described as 'medical'. After all, it might be argued that reproduction is fundamentally a natural, and not a medical, matter. Yet inevitably medical issues do become involved, whether one is considering, as does Rebecca Cook,[1] access to increased levels of maternal survival and health, or high technology problems, such as those posed by the capacity of medicine to separate social and gestational mothers.[2] The medical control of abortion, even that carried out on grounds which are traditionally described as 'social', and medicine's capacities to predict congenital defects, reinforce the medicalization of contraception, conception and childbirth. This is a worldwide phenomenon:

> Child-bearing and child-birth has come under male domination in the so-called developed world and increasingly, in the spread of Western medical practice and 'population programmes', in the developing.[3]

Legal and social process are thereby significantly affected by the input of orthodox medicine and the extent to which it is supported by law.

Medicine, then, has informed the social debate, contributed through education to at least the potential of changing sexual and reproductive patterns and influenced policy-makers and legislators. At least in the so-called developed world, problems can be identified and actively tackled by the dissemination of relevant information, gained from highly sophisticated orthodox medicine, whilst in other parts of the world the absence of access to that same information and those same sets of skills can be shown seriously to affect fundamental freedom and rights. To this extent, the positive involvement of medicine, technology and the state, in what is an essentially private aspect of personal liberty can be both desirable and autonomy-enhancing.

More threatening, however, to individual reproductive choices can be said to be the potential for non-voluntary or involuntary intervention in reproductive freedom, generated by factors external to the rights of the individual and his or her interest in reproductive choice, and which is, or can be, explained or justified by the involvement and superior knowledge of medicine and technology. In particular, 'scientific' knowledge and power can affect the rights of women, sometimes without their perception of this fact. As Davies, for example, notes:

> Not all feminists recognise that it is at the crossroads of female sexuality and biology, the bearing of children, that the bastion of male control is being fortified. More women may be entering the arena of public life, but with bizarre historical timing there is more control exerted over us in private life, particularly through obstetrics, by the increased use of technology. . . . The concentration on test-tube babies for the few, and the allocation of resources to infertility management in lieu of self-empowering health education are part of this same process.[4]

The history of reproductive freedom (or lack of it) is not divorced from either political influence or the impact of technological change.[5] In many significant ways the two have, in fact, combined to create an awesome juggernaut of apparent scientific certainty which has been used, whether or not deliberately, to ride over the interests, rights or freedoms of individuals caught in its path. Yet in matters of individual freedoms, and in situations which are directly concerned with human rights, it is not clear that political aspirations or technology should have such major influence. The debates surrounding new technological capacities in human reproduction are routinely couched in terms of morality, and certainly moral issues and values are involved. Equally, opposing instinctive or cultural opinions can be ultimately irreconcileable, even although all may be based on factual information as well as religious or moral views. In matters as private and as fundamental as reproductive freedom, we would do well to heed the following:

> In societies where respect for personal autonomy and for 'human rights' are fundamental moral principles the usual answer is that while people may reason with each other they must allow each other to come to their own moral decisions and to act accordingly provided

only that such action does not infringe upon the equal rights of others.[6]

Yet the history of reproductive choice scarcely leads to the conclusion that non-intervention, or respect for the position of others, is the norm.

This history continues to have relevance in the contemporary situation, although the nature of potential intervention may have been modified and the apparent need to insist on reproductive rights may have lost some of its sharp focus. At least, this is true in some parts of the world. The divide between the rich world and the poor world shows, however, the extent to which issues of reproductive choice can be polarized both within and between societies. Perhaps not surprisingly, in a book contributed to by those in the rich world, the focus of attention here has substantially been on the consequences of the dramatic technological impact on the pattern of human reproduction and the legal and ethical problems posed by them. Although the plight of the poor world is not entirely untouched, it is interesting to note the extent to which modern technological capacity seems to be leading the ethical debate and shaping the moral issues. In a sense, concentration of this sort can serve further to blur the nature of the debate and to disguise the character of the enterprise itself.

Whilst not denying that reproductive freedom has significance for both sexes, for the married and the unmarried, for the lesbian and the homosexual and for any resulting children, it remains crucial that any policy designed to expand or contract reproductive choice honestly confronts the fundamental point that the primary bearers of interests in human reproduction remain women, who generally carry the social, physical, psychological and practical burdens of childbearing and rearing. Whilst this may seem trite, it is possible for it to be forgotten as technological development alters the reproductive landscape and changes the ground rules. At the same time as technology permits some people access to reproductive choices which would otherwise have been denied, it can also involve the perceived need for a delicate balancing of other rights and interests, and can be used to limit freedoms. Moreover, it can entail that, ' . . . a normal female function [pregnancy and childbirth], which sometimes needs medical assistance, has come to be defined as defective and always in need of medical supervision.'[7]

These problems sometimes spill over into other aspects of reproductive freedom – such as the decision *not* to reproduce. For example, the capacity of modern medicine to keep some very premature babies alive has provided fuel for the fire of those who would seek to deny women real choice in pregnancy termination.

Equally, medical control of abortion has meant that terminations are carried out in certain ways and by specific means, which – in some countries at least – serve to sharpen the polarization of views by inevitably equating termination of a pregnancy with the death of a foetus.[8]

The fact that, at the moment, the United Kingdom Parliament is considering yet another attempt to limit the availability of abortion is closely linked to developments in postnatal intensive care. Indeed, the Bill's proposer has explained his case as being intimately linked to the right to life of the foetus.[9] Yet, an 18-week time limit on pregnancy termination would effectively add little to foetal rights, whilst simultaneously reducing maternal rights. The moment at which science declares a foetus to be viable (or at least potentially salvageable given an intensive and expensive medical input) can, as in this case, play a major role in defining the point at which women can lay claim to rights in this area.

Yet, it must be said, the issue is far wider than merely the capacities of medicine. Nonetheless, in the developed world at least, it could be argued that there is an increasing temptation to value other rights equally with those of women, or in some cases as being more important.[10] Moreover, although the position and the problems of women in the developing world may differ substantially from those of many women in the rich world, the practicalities of this distinction do not in themselves deny the essential similarities of women's claims and needs in respect of reproductive freedom. Although the debate in the rich world (or large parts of it) has switched to more esoteric and sophisticated matters, such as surrogacy, the 'rights' of the infertile and the 'rights' of the foetus, at root remain the central claims and interests of women to decide when, whether and how to reproduce.

Politics and reproduction

It is evident that reproductive practices have political significance. The very survival of the species depends on women bearing offspring and may indeed depend on the number of offspring produced, because of either under- or overpopulation. This means that total reproductive freedom, covering all aspects of reproductive choice from contraception to pregnancy termination to access to modern reproductive technology – whilst a goal for many women – is likely to remain unattainable. Gordon notes, for example, that '[b]irth control has always been regulated in some way. This is because birth control has consequences for two social issues crucial to overall social development: sexual activity and population size'.[11]

Equally, as Davies notes, social control may represent little more than the interests of one group or profession, or the short-term interests of the state – distancing the debate from the real interest bearers:

> The early commercial battles between the rubber industry and the chemical industry over the wombs of women must be remembered before contraception is awarded the status of liberator. Abortion policy, like contraception, is determined more by the national interest or the size of its labour or fighting force, than by woman's right to control the output of her own body. The interpretation of the 1967 Abortion Act, which effectively cut maternal mortality from illegal abortions and thereby improved the position of Britain in the international health league tables, is still the subjective decision of doctors.[12]

Moreover, when policies *do* develop which seem to be based on, or to encourage, the generation of rights for women, their motivation may be far from one which actively seeks to achieve this. This has significance for those to whom rights are apparently given, since motivation for reform which is not based on recognition of their fundamental rights may readily be changed by political, economic or social whim.

Political ambition may produce active and campaigning politicians with the impetus to adopt one political stance rather than another, and lead to an expansion or contraction of the right of others. As Luker[13] notes, the liberalization of California's abortion legislation came about (at the political level at least) partly as a result of some relatively new legislators seeking a political agenda by selecting new, but not (in their view) dangerous, issues on which to make a stand. Modification of this posture, however, may equally be facilitated by apparent shifts in 'public opinion' irrespective of the impact on those to whom the 'rights' are of crucial importance.

Political influence, in any society, is, of course, not uncommon. But, in matters of privacy, its impact can arguably be more invidious, pervasive and significant than in other areas of life. This is particularly clear when politicians use the language of morality to disguise uncritical acceptance of, or dependence on, a scientific or moral position whose terms are not shaped by those bearing the primary interests. This is not, of course, to suggest that there are no moral issues associated with matters of privacy, nor that politicians should inevitably be outlawed from expressing opinions on them, but rather to argue that it is imperative to remember the distinction between the use of moral discourse and morality itself. There *are* moral issues related to human reproductive practices, but the continual thrusting of matters of private liberty into the public arena often serves to generate the use of rights talk rather than facilitating the recognition and protection of the rights themselves. The rhetoric of morality can result in obfuscation of the fact that the motivation for intervention may be more pragmatic and less lofty than that dictated by morality itself.

Commentators have long noted and discussed the influence which the development of medical professionalism had on certain aspects of reproductive choice,[14] and the continuing influence which this (predominantly male) professional group has had on such matters.[15] Equally, legislators, judges and other influential groups are increasingly aware of the rudimentaries of technological capacity in reproductive matters, and better informed on the extent to which their public attitude may gain or lose them points. Just as it is widely recognized that the political colour of the US Supreme Court can make significant changes to the liberties accorded to the average citizen, so the politicization of debates about intensely personal matters can lead to subversion of the fundamental issues.

As Luker,[16] for example, suggests, the debate between 'pro-life' and 'pro-choice' activists in the abortion question is essentially irreconcileable. The two sides can take the same information, but interpret it in an entirely different way, or weight each informational item quite differently. Where politicians and lawyers seek to adopt a conciliatory position they are, therefore, essentially doomed to failure, and yet substantial political pressures may be brought to bear by either, usually both, of these opposing groups. Thus, although it has been claimed that the fundamentals of reproductive freedoms are the rights of *women*, the perceived need to tailor political views to enhance the opportunity for political victory serves to deny, or at least to minimize, their significance.

Women's rights are thereby confronted with an impressively armed enemy. Political interests, medical pressures and ultimately legal control may serve to ensure that many women are effectively disenfranchised on this issue; judged or deskilled by superior 'knowledge' in this most intimate of choices. Recent cases in the UK have served to demonstrate the extent to which reproductive freedom is now seen, at least in respect of certain groups, as a legitimate interest of the law, backed by medical judgement. Decisions to sterilize (and in one case also to abort) young mentally handicapped women,[17] have been justified on the grounds that they would be unable to parent, on medical opinion that pregnancy would be distressing, or on the view that, in any event, the women would not miss the capacity to breed because of their intellectual limitations.[18] Moreover, lifestyle has been taken, when the decision is made by doctors, to be a plausible reason for denying access to

modern reproductive techniques.[19] Those who believe that legal
and political influences are no longer significant issues and that
the contemporary attitude to reproductive choice is a liberal one,
perhaps even one which gives women too much choice, should
study these cases carefully.

Technology and reproduction

It is of course possible to disguise a political agenda as merely being
a response to technological knowledge and development. In a world
dominated by rapid, and often astonishing, technological advance,
technology itself becomes a useful tool in the debate. If seen as a
value free enterprise (as it often seems to be) then it plays an
apparently innocent role in modifying society, opportunities and
attitudes. Yet:

> When we talk of technology, we are not only talking about a product
> or a process (a home computer or an automated factory, for example)
> but also about a whole set of ideas and values that go into the design,
> making and use of such a product or process.[20]

Indeed, even where the moral dilemmas posed by technology are
overt and unavoidable, the deployment of technology can be
presented as nonetheless only the concern of those who understand
it. Thus, the capacity of medicine to keep alive severely damaged
infants has raised the moral dilemma of whether or not such efforts
should be made. Although clearly a matter of general social concern,
British courts at least have been reluctant to interfere in the
professional decisions of doctors – a tacit (and in some cases quite
explicit) handing over of moral and practical authority to those who
profess the technical expertise, *because* of their possession of that
expertise.[21]

Further, as has been noted, medicine's capacity to keep premature babies alive much earlier nowadays has provided ammunition
for those who oppose abortion to argue that foetuses of the same
gestational age should not be aborted. Whilst understandable, and
indeed not inevitably irrelevant, the fundamental issue is however
ignored by such an approach. If medical science is developing in
such a way as to lower the age of 'viability', then simple adoption
of viability as a criterion for pregnancy termination has far-reaching
and serious implications for the rights of women. If by some miracle
(no stranger to contemporary medicine) the time at which foetuses
can be preserved *extra utero* became, for example, 12 weeks, should
this be taken as evidence that abortions could only be performed,

say, at 10 weeks, so that – given the two weeks for a margin of error – every foetus can be saved? In other words, are foetal rights inevitably paramount? And if they are, how can this be reconciled with a legal system which simultaneously turns a blind eye to, or actively refuses to criticise, a practice of killing (or letting die) fully developed foetuses (now called babies)? And what are the problems for women inherent in such a view?

The use of technology is by no means an uncommon feature of the history of intervention in reproductive choice. The early eugenicists relied on elementary genetic knowledge (and specu-lation) to influence significantly the pattern of reproductive free-doms in many countries – notably in the first half of this century. Scientific claims apparently dominated social direction, but of course they also disguised, under the veneer of value-free scientific knowledge, a political agenda which was anything but value-free. Nor has the situation necessarily changed merely because tech-nology is more sophisticated, because the public is apparently better informed and because we live in an apparently more liberal age.

Rather, it could be argued that technology is a better friend of the political agenda in contemporary society. Because it is so far removed from the experience and understanding of the average person, its hidden values are more readily disguised, and its interpretation more easily dominated by those who manipulate it. The opportunity for an élite group to maximize social influence is, therefore, potentially enhanced. Control of reproductive technology permits the making of 'professional' judgements which can shape the debate as a whole. Two situations spring to mind immediately. To return briefly to the issue of abortion, it has already been pointed out that, if the capacity of technology to define and redefine viability is taken as a moral or legal yardstick for the time at which preg-nancies can legally be terminated, then logically this could continue to reduce women's freedoms to make choices. Indeed, it seems to be assumed that the potential to keep aborted foetuses alive, had they been born prematurely rather than aborted, is a sound reason for lowering the legal time limit for abortion. Clearly, however, this is by no means the only option available, but the fact that it is the one most routinely canvassed might be thought to say something about the motivation behind efforts to reduce the time limit.

What, for example, would be the position if women seeking terminations at a stage where the foetus medically had some pros-pect of survival were presented with the option of a pregnancy termination which did not inevitably result in the death of the foetus? It is, of course, not possible to answer this question defini-tively, but the fact that it is almost never broached seems somewhat strange if the aim really is to balance rights. The medical termination of later pregnancies seems, in fact, to be designed to ensure the death of the foetus, but from where did this moral warrant come?[22] It is equally plausible to argue that the woman seeks merely to relieve herself of the pregnancy, but that – where the foetus may be salvageable – she does not necessarily intend its death. In fact, of course, and regardless of the actual wishes of women, in English law at least:

> . . . it is only by ensuring that the child is not born alive, following an abortion, that a doctor can be certain that his conduct could not under any circumstances amount to the offence of child murder.[23]

Whose interests, then, are represented and protected by these practices? Certainly, there seems to be no direct advertance to the rights or interests of women, whose position in society may be seriously denigrated by the perception of sectors of the public that *they* intend child destruction – a view which provides ammunition for those who would seek to minimize women's rights in this area.

The fact that staff in hospitals are distressed by, on the one hand doing all in their power to save the life of a wanted foetus born prematurely at, say, 26 weeks, and on the other destroying foetuses of the same age in abortions is often used to show the iniquity of abortion. However, it could equally be used to demand evaluation of the underlying *medical* choices which are made without reference to the women whose rights are vulnerable to public perception of the result of the techniques adopted by medicine in pregnancy termination. In other words, women are accused of essentially killing babies because medicine has elected to interpret pregnancy termination as necessarily involving foetal destruction. Adopting a different perspective on the rights and interests involved in pregnancy termination could serve to shift the focus of the debate. Some commentators, for example, would argue that the debate is better and more appropriately conducted in alternative terms – for example, the woman's right to 'self-ownership'. In line with this approach, the mother could still vindicate her right to self-ownership, even where viability is reached, by ejecting the unwanted foetus in a manner consonant with saving its life.[24]

Now it may be the case that, even if women were consulted, they would prefer that a foetus did not survive, but one thing is absolutely clear and that is that they are not given the opportunity to decide. As a result of this, they become in a very real sense the victims of medical decisions – victims whose fundamental freedoms are restricted by their inability to participate fully in a debate which, it can be argued, in any event is conducted on inappropriate lines and within a misleading framework.

Indeed, the suggestion that questions of women's rights are inadequately considered in this issue is also reinforced by the deceptions which colour the current attempts to reform the Abortion laws in the UK. As was noted earlier, it is said that the reason for seeking to amend the Abortion Act is intimately connected to the desire to protect foetal life. Yet reducing the time limit to 18 weeks effectively ensures the death of the foetus. Moreover, the Bill's sponsor has indicated that he would not be entirely and unalterably opposed to extending the time limit for termination in those cases – currently the focus of much public and media attention – where the termination is inevitably delayed by the need to test for foetal handicap at a certain stage in the pregnancy.[25] If all foetal life is sacred, then why should younger ones not be, and on what grounds are handicapped ones not? In other words, this reform, as all others, fails to challenge abortion techniques and to tackle the real issues, and is no more than a thinly disguised attempt to restrict women's rights. By couching the debate in these terms, women also become scapegoats. Not only are other, unconnected, people permitted to reduce their capacity for choices, but they are branded as 'child-killers'.

The other example relates to more modern problems. The development of *in vitro* fertilization techniques has generated considerable public interest and controversy. One issue on which much energy has been focused is that which concerns the fate of 'spare' embryos. Can or should such embryos be used for experimental purposes? Do the donors of the genetic material have any rights or choices over this?

It might plausibly be argued, and indeed is argued by many supporters of technical advance that, if a spare embryo has been created, and is not to be implanted, it can scarcely be worse to experiment on it before it is destroyed than simply to destroy it. The embryo can feel no pain, the research is conducted by professionals in appropriate settings and with sufficient dignity, and in any event the benefits of embryo research may be huge in terms of, for example, the prediction and perhaps the elimination of many genetic handicaps.[26] A plausible argument indeed, but one which has nonetheless failed to endear itself to large sections of the public.

Whilst the debate about embryo experiments is not strictly relevant here, it is raised to make one specific point. The whole IVF programme is intimately linked in many people's minds with embryo experimentation, because it is practice to create (potentially) spare embryos. The capacity of that programme to facilitate reproductive choice for women (and men) is tainted by the fear of immoral experimentation on embryos. Yet, the creation of 'spare'

embryos, whilst accepted medical practice, is by no means an inevitable concommitant of IVF. It is rather a practice developed by the
medical profession on grounds which, whilst undoubtedly
designed to be in the interests of their patients, may yet serve to
restrict their rights. Doubtless it is preferable that women should
not have to go through the (albeit relatively minimal) risks of
repeated laparoscopies, and doubtless also implantation of a
number of embryos may increase the likelihood of establishing a
pregnancy, but if the outcome of using this technique is the creation
of antipathy to the entire programme, then perhaps the best interests of present and future patients are not in fact served by current
practice. Again, however, it is clear that women, who remain the
central characters, are uninvolved in the relevant decisions.

Whither women's rights?

Scientific advances and technological developments may enhance
liberty but they also have the capacity to restrict it. This may be
done in a number of ways, and in the debates about reproduction
those who manipulate technology can be accused of having in part
posed unnecessary problems of a moral nature, and perhaps even
of defeating their own interest in pursuing the scientific path on
which they have embarked. 'Public opinion' can be a powerful
tool, however speculative its content, and 'public opinion' is both
depended on and shaped by these kinds of medical choices, since
the public is unlikely to be aware that there *is* an alternative, and
that some practices which seem to pose moral dilemmas are not
the only possible way of doing things. In areas of great sensitivity,
and deeply felt anxiety, the Warnock Committee,[27] for example,
used precisely this device – of appealing to 'public opinion' – to
bolster conclusions which they clearly wanted to reach. Inevitably,
and whatever the state of public opinion in advance of the publication of this Report, their conclusions have subsequently been
absorbed into the public consciousness.

On the other hand, the people whose rights and desires are
frustrated by overreaction or radical intervention are those for
whom childrearing is a priority. The classic example in many ways
is the debate over surrogacy,[28] which a majority of the Warnock
Committee sought to outlaw.[29] In this case, however, the UK
government's recent White Paper[30] is more cautious, and more
closely allied to views such as those expressed by Winslade,[31] who
concluded that, in view of lack of evidence of harm and the moral
confusion surrounding surrogacy:

The law should . . . play neither a reactionary nor a revolutionary role. This means that the practice [of surrogacy] should be legally permitted but cautiously regulated, and morally tolerated but carefully scrutinised.[32]

This is not to say that public debate or opinion (if we could actually identify it) on matters of morality is inappropriate or irrelevant, nor to suggest that there are no issues in human reproduction which can ever be compared with the rights of women. However, once we admit that women are the primary bearers of rights, then it is essential that any recommendation or law which is designed to restrict such rights is thoroughly and openly justified on grounds which are more than simply the distaste – real or assumed – of some sections of the community. This is another situation where we should aspire to the *use* of morality rather than merely dressing our own prejudice in its *language*. Nowhere is this need more clear than in the case of what has come to be known as 'surrogacy for convenience'.

The woman who chooses parenthood without pregnancy, for reasons which are personally valid, is condemned or treated with suspicion, just as is the woman who makes the converse decision – pregnancy without parenthood. The combination of legal sanction and medical monopoly permits value-laden decisions about, for example, fitness for parenting, and tends to be restrictive rather than permissive. In any event, even if the Warnock Committee is right to argue that the majority of public opinion is offended by certain reproductive practices, it is not clear why the individual who feels no such abhorrence should be bound by this. In the global situation the fact that A is upset by B's choice seems scarcely a sufficiently weighty reason to deny B fundamental liberties. But it is not unusual to use women's reproductive capacities as a ground for maintaining a facade of social stability which defeats the claims of women to equality. Freedom of choice in reproduction might equally present a threat to accepted wisdom as to the nature of acceptable female roles and behaviour. Johnsen, for example, notes that:

State and social regulations based on women's ability to bear children have created and reinforced separate and unequal sex-segregated spheres in our society. Reproductive differences between the sexes have served as the justification for excluding women from the paid labor force and the political process and confining them to the private sphere of the home and family where they depended on their husbands and fathers for economic and social status.[33]

The traditional pattern of intrusion into women's (and sometimes men's) reproductive rights has taken a further, and sinister, turn in the recent past. Where technology creates, with state resources, facilities for the artificial creation of fertility (or at least the circumvention of inability to parent) amongst the 10–15 per cent of the population thought to be infertile,[34] the manner in which these resources are allocated must be closely scrutinized if prejudice and untested values are not to dominate decision-making. Yet, to date, little seems to have been done to evaluate the bases on which such scarce resources are morally to be allocated,[35] even though they may challenge our very understanding of 'personhood' and our tolerance of different habits, priorities or lifestyles.

Yet, whether or not we have thought through the moral principles underlying choice, the reality is nonetheless that such choices are currently being made. In the English High Court recently, a former prostitute lost her appeal against removal from an artificial reproduction programme on grounds that, because of her lifestyle, she was an unsuitable person to become a parent.[36] That she was consistently lied to as to the reasons for this removal is bad enough, but that the court expressed the view that, in taking this decision, neither the consultant in charge of the case nor the hospital's Infertility Service Ethical Committee 'had ultimately acted unreasonably or unlawfully'[37] gives rise to even more concern.

'Fitness for parenting' is a concept which defies definition on any basis which could satisfy an unbiased moral opinion. But its use has, nonetheless, become increasingly prevalent. Just as the cases of *T. v. T. and Anor.*[38] and *Re B (Sterilisation)*[39] overtly used impressions about fitness for parenting in reaching their conclusion that sterilization of mentally handicapped young women could be authorized by the courts,[40] so too may the infertile find themselves tacitly assessed for parenting in a way which permits value-laden and untestable criteria to be used by those who may be good scientists but of uncertain qualification in such speculative matters as parenting competence. In any event, is this the kind of decision that anyone should be taking, when the result of taking it is the denial of a fundamental human right?

Moreover, assessment of 'fitness for parenting' does not stop there. Recent trends have demonstrated an increasing willingness on the part of the law to intervene in the relationship between the pregnant woman and foetus, by the device of contrasting maternal and foetal 'rights'.[41] Attempts to make unborn children wards of court in an effort to impose standards of behaviour on pregnant women, whether or not the pregnancy was natural, have so far failed in the English courts,[42] but that the issue is raised at all is a matter of concern. Although these devices have been unsuccessful pre-birth, they have been more successful immediately following the birth of the child. A mentally handicapped couple recently faced the full apparatus of the law's successful attempts to have their child removed immediately following birth, on the grounds that they would not be 'fit' parents. On 25 January 1988, the Birmingham High Court confirmed that the child should remain in care since the parents were deemed incapable of looking after it.[43]

The movement to force women into behavioural patterns during pregnancy – perhaps even before it – depends on the elevation of the foetus to the status of an entity with rights which are capable of taking priority over those of women to choose their lifestyle. Recent cases where maternal and foetal rights have been contrasted, however, show the dangerous potential of viewing reproduction in this way. Johnsen,[44] comments on some of these problems with reference to the case of Pamela Rae Stewart, who was arrested and charged with causing her son's death by, amongst other things, failing to obtain adequate medical care in the course of her pregnancy. Although the case was subsequently dismissed, Johnsen suggests that one of the reasons for the current plethora of attempts to constrain pregnant women through the use of the criminal law in the USA is the fact that '[t]hough manifested thus far in a haphazard, even unthinking manner, the clear trend has been to expand "fetal rights" at the expense of pregnant women'.[45] Indeed, in California, the scene of the Pamela Rae Stewart case, Senator Ed Royce remains committed to the introduction of a Bill which would include foetuses in child protection legislation,[46] thus reinforcing the current trend for court-ordered intervention in pregnancy and childbirth.[47] As the *Guardian* noted, '[a] woman's rights to privacy, autonomy and freedom from assault have been enshrined in British common law and the American constitution. Now those rights are in question.'[48] In reality, neither British or US law has ever shown itself committed to, or adept at, protecting them. The apparent priority currently given to the future upbringing of a child, and to the production of 'normal' babies – even the Alton Bill would apparently concede the latter – has generated an atmosphere of coercion rather than education. As has been noted:

> Reports are accumulating from all over the U.S. on judicial coercion of pregnant women. These include a number of court orders for caesarean sections and intrauterine transfusions against the will of the women concerned, and the detention during pregnancy of at least one teenager who 'lacked the ability' to seek pre-natal care.[49]

These coercive activities continue even in the face of the legal problems of either stipulating the content of any offence committed by pregnant women or providing sanctions for breach. It would be extremely difficult to create an offence that was suitable unless it was one of strict liability, since, as Fortim notes,[50] it is at the earliest stages of pregnancy that damage is most likely to occur. Just how it could be established that the woman had the necessary intention to harm the foetus, for example in situations where she may not even have been aware that she was pregnant, it is difficult to envisage. And what would be reasonable or workable sanctions?

It is paradoxical that when the thalidomide tragedy occurred in the UK,[51] the law was castigated for a lack of clarity on the question of whether or not a chld born alive, but damaged pre-birth, had a right to raise an action, yet two decades later, the foetus' interests and rights seem to dominate the law's concerns in this area. The relatively innocent retrospective recognition of foetal 'rights' where damage is negligently caused pre-birth or pre-conception may unfortunately, and unwittingly, have served in part to legitimate wider intrusion into maternal rights by apparently recognizing foetal rights. This is particularly poignant in English law, which on the one hand has recently held that it is legitimate in care proceedings to look at a mother's behaviour in the course of a pregnancy,[52] but which refuses to authorize a child to sue its mother for compensation where that behaviour has caused handicap.[53] The paradox in part lies in the fact that the right to sue was considered inappropriate because of its potential adverse effects on the mother–child relationship,[54] yet the same behaviour is now increasingly used to remove the child from his or her mother. What could have a more direct and detrimental impact on the mother–child relationship than this?

Conclusions

An examination of many of the issues discussed in this book shows the extent to which the pattern of interest in reproductive choice has come full circle. From the debates of the last century over what is now regarded as relatively routine (for example, access to contraception) to concerns about modern reproductive techniques and the quality of life, certain constants remain. The medicalization of pregnancy and childbirth, and the political and legal controls on access to reproductive freedoms, continue to hold the centre of the debate at a distance from those whom it actively and actually concerns. Women's choices about when, whether, where and how to breed continue to be circumscribed and delimited by the prejudices and interests of others. As has been said, ' . . . in the allocation of resources which define how we function from birth to death, here and in the so-called underdeveloped countries the common denominator is the lack of equal control by women'.[55] Legal intervention, when closely analysed, tends also to be restrictive rather than permissive.

The fact that women's fertility (or lack of it) has traditionally been seen as something which others have a legitimate voice, has served to suggest that the issue is not a question of women's rights and freedoms, but is rather one on which the morals or moral discourse of others have a legitimate bearing. Thus, it becomes plausible to discuss and analyse biological functions in terms of competing rights and interests – even where (as with the abortion debate) the rights and interests of the person most directly involved might, as a consequence of this analysis, be denied or defeated. The capacity to control reproductive technology may then be taken as a sufficient condition for decision-making dominance.

In conclusion, therefore, it is argued that it is important to bear in mind that – despite the tone of some debates – reproduction (or not) is not *in se* a matter of morality, and that where it is, the moral questions and concerns can be separated from the fact of reproduction (or not). Moreover, the nature of any consequential moral debate may be thoroughly disparate depending on whether or not one is concerned with the rich or the poor world. For example, the struggle for antenatal care and access to reproductive control, which forms the primary issue of concern for the poor world,[56] is not generally problematic in the rich world.

Control over (primarily female) reproductive practices has emerged as an aspiration of many states and political and legal ideologies. Its exposure as a means of exploiting certain groups has been successfully conducted in a number of countries particularly in the course of the twentieth century. However, the denunciation of wholesale compulsory sterilization campaigns, or the dismissal of certain views as mere religious fanaticism, should not disguise the potential for the reintroduction and reassertion of discredited and distasteful limitations on the liberty and privacy of the individual, by sheltering them behind a technological screen.

Many individuals stand to lose such reproductive freedom as they have if the elements of the reproduction debate are not separated, analysed and considered without prejudice. The rights of women have dominated this discussion, but it needs little imagination to identify others whose rights can be infringed by value-laden decisions taken by politicians, lawyers and the controllers of technology. Other groups against whom discrimination is already not unusual, such as homosexuals, can equally be victims. As Hanscombe notes:

. . . cruel and heartless lobbying from powerful religious and political quarters – aimed against the human rights of adult homosexual women and men – is ongoing, despite its lack of scientific objectivity. Such pressure is also richly funded.[57]

Technologizing reproduction, and thereby reshaping the moral questions which *are* involved, means, however, that an array of arguments may be produced to limit the availability of resources to groups whose rights to reproduce are already regarded as nugatory. As Hanscombe further notes:

> There are no data – scientific, psychological or social – which could support the thesis that homosexual people should not have the right to reproduce and to bring up their children. There are only differing opinions and prejudices, which are not capable of sustaining the rigorous intellectual analysis upon which any given body of knowledge must rest.[58]

Equally, the unmarried, whatever their sexual preference, may find themselves described as a non-group for the purposes of access to the parenting opportunities offered by modern technology. As Singer and Wells note;

> To restrict this treatment [IVF] to married couples would be a precedent, since no other medical treatment is legally restricted to only a sub-class of those who need it (need here being demonstrated by willingness to go through a gruelling regimen).[59]

It is technology which, in many cases, has forced consideration of the unstated and untested assumptions upon which limitation of personal freedom is based, but equally it is the controllers of technology who ultimately decide whether the matter is an appropriate one for public debate, and who in any event can allocate resources in the guise of professional rather than personal decision-making. That a number of speculative, and perhaps unacceptable, criteria are used seems uncontestable, yet as Harris says:

> . . . in the absence of a general and fair scheme for scrutinising all parents and without a clear conception of what constitutes fitness, it is both invidious and disturbing when chance leads to a particular parent being effectively declared unfit in the absence of, and in advance of, any palpable evidence. If low IQ or inadequate housing or even the presence of elderly and perhaps unsupportive people were disqualifying conditions for parenthood, the world would quickly become depopulated. This might well be a good thing, but it is far from clear that such a policy should be initiated by general practitioners and even health visitors on their own say-so.[60]

This perspective has equal relevance in relation to choices *not* to parent.

In postulating one solution or another to these perceived or real dilemmas it is argued here that it is vital to bear in mind the need to address the basic issues rather than being seduced into considering peripheral ones. The publicization of essentially private matters may often, therefore, be unncessary. Accepting the essentially private nature of such choices renders them less vulnerable to exploitation by those who have different political, religious or social perspectives and whose interest in the private behaviour of other individuals is arguably of tenuous legitimacy. Moreover, it must not be assumed that either technology or those who use it, are value-free in what they do. It seems not unreasonable to suggest that the person most directly involved should be entitled to information, and to participation in, if not domination of, decision-making. Neither the sophistication of a technique nor the esoteric nature of professional jargon should be used to validate a claim that the individual involved is not equipped to make a decision.

The paradox for the moment is that the real moral debate – that which concerns the rights of those who have legitimate interests in contraception, pregnancy, childbirth and access to modern reproductive technology – seems to have been circumvented by the issues which are peripheral: for example, the techniques medically selected for terminating pregnancies, viability, embryo experiments, foetal 'rights', sexual behaviour and sexual preference. Our values and perspectives will remain uninformed and ill thought-out until these marginal trees are thinned to enable examination of the wood.

Notes

1   See Chapter 8 *supra*.
2   See Chapter 7, *supra*.
3   Davies, J., 'Women and health' in Ashworth,G., and Bonnerjea, L. (eds), *The Invisible Decade: U.K. Women and the U.N. Decade 1976–1985*, Aldershot, Gower, 1985, p. 94.
4   Loc. cit., note 3, *supra*, p. 85.
5   For discussion, cf. Gordon, L., *Woman's Body, Woman's Right*, Harmondsworth, Penguin, 1977; McLean, S. A. M., 'The right to reproduce' in Campbell, T., Goldberg, D., McLean, S. A. M. and Mullen, T. (eds), *Human Rights: From Rhetoric to Reality*, Oxford, Basil Blackwell, 1986.
6   '*In Vitro* fertilisation' (editorial), **9** *Journal of Medical Ethics*, 187, 1983, 188.
7   Davies, *loc. cit.* note 3, *supra*, p. 94.
8   It is worth noting that David Steel's Bill, which became the Abortion Act 1967, was less emotively entitled the Medical Termination of Pregnancy Bill. For a discussion of legal liability in pregnancy termination see Skegg, P. D. G., *Law, Ethics and Medicine*, Oxford, Clarendon Press, 1984, ch. 1.

9   Abortion (Amendment) Bill 1987. See, for example, almost daily reports in the press during January 1988. In answer to a parliamentary debate on his Bill, Mr David Alton argued that, given the ' "gigantic steps in medical technology", . . . it was now incumbent on MPs to review the balance between claimed rights and responsibilities'.: *Guardian*, 23 January 1988. For a more detailed discussion of the abortion debate, see Chapter 3, *supra*.

10 See, for discussion, Johnsen, D., 'A new threat to pregnant women's autonomy'. **17** *Hastings Center Report*, 33, 1987.

11 Gordon, *op. cit.*, note 5 *supra*, p. 3.

12 Loc. cit., note 3 *supra*, p. 93.

13 Luker, K., *Abortion and the Politics of Motherhood*, University of California Press, 1984.

14 Cf. Mohr, J. C., *Abortion in America*, New York, Oxford University Press, 1978.

15 An influence which means that medical support and approval are generally required before access to pregnancy termination, although in some countries this is limited to the later pregnancy termination only. For discussion, see Freeman, M. D. A., 'The lesson Alton's supporters refuse to learn', *Guardian*, 22 January 1988.

16 Luker, op. cit., note 13 *supra*.

17 For further discussion, see Chapter 6 *supra*.

18 *T. v. T. & Anor The Times*, 11 July 1987; *Re B* [1987] 2 All ER 206 (CA); *The Times*, 17 March 1987 (HL).

19 For discussion, see 'Ex-prostitute says doctor unfair on test-tube baby', *Guardian*, 21 October 1987.

20 Zmroczek, C., Henwood, F. and Wyatt, S., 'Women and technology' in Ashworth and Bonnerjea, op. cit., note 3 *supra*, p. 121.

21 Cf. *R* v. *Arthur*, *The Times*, 6 November 1981, where the decision of a doctor (and parents) not to treat a handicapped infant resulted in the doctor's eventual acquittal on a charge of attempted murder. For discussion of the issues involved, see Chapter 5, *supra*.

22 Skegg, op. cit., note 8, *supra*, provides at least one legal reason for the adoption of techniques which ensure that foetuses do not survive – a reason which, however, has nothing to do with the women concerned.

23 Cf. Skegg, *op. cit.*, note 8 *supra*, p. 26.

24 Cf. Paul, E. F. and Paul, J., 'Self-ownership, abortion and infanticide' **5** *Journal of Medical Ethics* 133, 1979.

25 See, for example, David Alton's response to parliamentary questioning on this matter, reported, for example, in the *Guardian*, 23 January 1988.

26 For discussion of the pros and cons of embryo research, see *Report of the Committee of Inquiry Into Human Fertilisation and Embryology* (Warnock Report), Cmnd. 9314/1984.

27 *Supra cit.*, note 26.

28 For further discussion, see Chapter 7, *supra*; for an alternative view, see Roberts, S., 'Warnock and surrogate motherhood: sentiment or argument?' in Byrne, P. (ed.), *Rights and Wrongs in Medicine*, Oxford University Press, (for the King's Fund, London), 1986.

29 Loc. cit., note 26, *supra* para 8.19: 'We recommend that it be provided by statute that all surrogacy arrangements are illegal contracts and therefore unenforceable in the courts.'

30 In para 75, the White Paper leaves the door open to the possibility of developing non-commercial surrogacy services ' . . . if it were concluded that, for example, non-commercial surrogacy services should be brought within the framework of the law.'

31 Winslade, W. J., 'Surrogate mothers: private right or public wrong?' 7 *Journal of Medical Ethics* 153, 1981.
32 Loc. cit., note 31, *supra* p. 153.
33 Loc. cit., note 10, *supra*, p. 38.
34 For further discussion, see Chapter 2, *supra*.
35 For a discussion of resource allocation in medicine, see McLean, S. A. M. and Maher, G., *Medicine, Morals and the Law*, Aldershot, Gower, 1983 (reprinted 1985), ch. 10.
36 Cf. report in the *Guardian*, 27 October 1987.
37 Id.
38 *Supra cit.*, note 18.
39 *Re B (Sterilisation)* [1987] 2 All ER 206 (CA); *The Times*, 17 March 1987.
40 For further discussion, see Chapter 6, *supra*.
41 For discussion, see Johnsen, *loc. cit.*, note 10, *supra*.
42 Cf. *Guardian*, 18 January 1988 and 5 February 1988.
43 *Guardian*, 26 January 1988.
44 Johnsen, loc cit., note 10, *supra*.
45 Ibid., p. 35.
46 Cf. report in the *Guardian*, 22 December 1987.
47 For discussion, see Kolder, U. E. B. Gallagher, J., and Parsons, M. T., 'Court-ordered obstetrical interventions', **316** *New England Journal of Medicine*, 1192, 1987.
48 *Guardian*, 12 December 1987.
49 Id.
50 Fortin, J. E. S., 'Legal Protection for the unborn child' **51** *Modern Law Review*, 54, 1988.
51 For a full and excellent discussion, see Teff, H. and Munro, C., *Thalidomide: The Legal Aftermath*, London, Saxon House, 1976.
52 *D.* v. *Berkshire C.C.* [1987] 1 All ER 20.
53 Congenital Disabilities (Civil Liability) Act 1976. In Scotland, a child has the right to sue either parent: *Young* v. *Rankin* 1934 SC 499.
54 Cf. Report of the (English) Law Commission, *Report on Injuries to Unborn Children* Cmnd. 5709, 1974.
55 Davies, loc. cit., note 3 *supra*, p. 85.
56 See Chapter 8, *supra*.
57 Manscombe, G., 'The right to lesbian parenthood', **9** *Journal of Medical Ethics* 133 1983, p. 135.
58 Ibid.; this assertion seems to be borne out further by research undertaken by Golumbok and Rust: see Golumbok, S. and Rust, J., 'The Warnock Report and single women: what about the children?', **12** *Journal of Medical Ethics*, 182, 1986, 185, where they note: 'Whether or not children born to lesbian mothers by AID or IVF are more likely to show atypical psychosexual development can only be determined by direct studies. However, the evidence that exists so far about the development of the handful of children who were raised in such families from birth, does not indicate any cause for concern.'
59 Singer, P. and Wells, D., '*In vitro* Fertilisation – the major issues; **9** *Journal of Medical Ethics* 192, 1983, 195.
60 Harris, J., 'Commentary' **9** *Journal of Medical Ethics*, 222, 1983, 223.

Index